Controlling Chronic Pain

CONNIE PECK is a Senior Lecturer in the Department of
Psychology at La Trobe University. She was born in the
United States and received her Ph.D from the University of
Wisconsin in 1974. Subsequently, she worked as a clinical
psychologist at the University of Washington Medical School
in the Department of Rehabilitation Medicine with patients
suffering pain and with other chronically ill and disabled
patients. Since going to Australia in 1977, Dr Peck has
continued her research into the management of chronic pain.
She has also been active in multidisciplinary research into
the management of post-operative pain at the Royal Southern
Memorial Hospital, Victoria.

Dr Peck is a member of the International Association for
the Study of Pain. She is the author of numerous articles
dealing with chronic pain and its treatment, and is co-author
of the book *Problems in Pain* (1980).

Controlling Chronic Pain

A Self-help Guide

Connie Peck

Fontana/Collins

First published in Australia by
Fontana Paperbacks, Sydney, 1982
Published in Great Britain, with Foreword by
Patrick Wall and various revisions, in 1985
by Fontana Paperbacks, 8 Grafton Street, London W1X 3LA

Copyright © Connie Peck 1982

Made and printed in Great Britain by
William Collins Sons & Co. Ltd, Glasgow

Contents

Foreword by Patrick D. Wall   ix

Preface   1

1   No, You're Not a Hypochondriac   3

2   The Chronic Pain Trap   10
The Medication Trap   10
The Take It Easy Trap   14
The Depression Trap   17
The Complaint-Resentment-Guilt Trap   18

3   Analysing What Chronic Pain
      Has Done to Your Life   24
Information Collecting on Current Activity   30
Information Collecting on Potential Activities   33
Information Collecting on How You Complain   37

4   Your Doctor and You   39

5   How to Resume More Normal Activity   46
Your Exercise Programme Contract   50
Graphing Your Progress   51

How to Select Rewards and Punishment   52
Increasing Walking   55
Increasing Sitting Time   66
Stair Climbing   70
Increasing Ability to Ride In or Drive a Car   73
Increasing Other Exercises   78
Increasing Housework   79
Increasing Other Types of Work Tolerance   84

6 Fighting Off the Depression of Chronic Pain   89
Learning to Like Yourself Better   90
Minimizing Unpleasant Experiences   95
Maximizing Pleasant Experiences   98
Maximizing Mastery Over the Environment   107

7 Controlling the Pain Killers   111

8 What to Do and What Not to Do
    When You Are in Pain   126

9 How You, the Family, Can Help   134
Over-protective Family Pattern   135
Isolation and Denial of the Problem   137
Pain as a Learned Response   139
The Maladaptive Family Learning Patterns   140
How to Change Maladaptive
    Family Learning Patterns   141

10 Preventing Pain   153
Forehead Tension   154
Jaw Tension   155
Neck and Shoulder Tension   156
Practising Relaxation   158
Biofeedback   159

11   **Recognizing and Solving Other Problems
         Which May Aggravate Pain   161**
     Sexual Problems   163
     Marital or Relationship Problems   166
     General Difficulty in Relating to Others   168
     Failure to Live Up to Expectations   170
     An Unhappy Job Situation   172
     Alcohol Problems   176
     Litigation   178
     Tension   180

12   **Maintaining Your Progress   183**

     Further Reading—For General Readers   189

     References—For Professional Readers   195

     **Appendix: Directory of Pain
         Clinics   202**

     Index   208

Foreword

Two hundred years ago, the curative power of medicine was minimal. Good people, doctors, nurses and those wise in the ways of life and death gathered around the patient. They tried their best to control unpleasant symptoms while nature took its course. They used every means at their disposal from pills to prayers, from massage to mumbo-jumbo. If the method worked, they went on using it without any embarrassment about their not having a scientific explanation for what they were doing.

A hundred years ago, modern medicine and surgery were being born. Doctors and patients set their sights on two clear targets. First, a single diagnosis of the cause of the disease. Second, a treatment which would cure. While making admirable progress for some patients towards these two targets, they reasonably rejected halfway measures such as the treatment of symptoms which did not attack the fundamental cause of the condition. The phrase 'mere symptomatic treatment' was used as synonymous with bad medicine. The splendid advances have not been uniform in achieving universal diagnosis or cure. For example, no one in the world understands the origin of the great majority of low back pains.

Controlling Chronic Pain

It is true that a fortunate minority can be precisely diagnosed as having a slipped disc which responds to surgery. This leaves a majority in real pain but without a rational diagnosis. In another sadly large group of patients, a very exact diagnosis is all too apparent, such as osteoarthritis or cancer, but no fundamental cure is yet available. In the exciting developments of this century, we have tended to neglect the symptoms of those unfortunate enough to have a disease which has so far eluded diagnosis or has no cure.

This period of neglect is ending. In an initiative started in America by Professor J. J. Bonica, the concept of a pain clinic has developed. Here ideally all available skills are brought together to try to avoid the morale-destroying progress of the patient from one occasionally successful specialist to another. In Britain, the hospice movement was revived by Dame Cicely Saunders with an addition of the best of modern medicine to the old arts of care and comforting. At the same time, there has been a change of attitude to pain itself and to its mechanisms in which Professor Melzack from Canada and I have played some part. It is now clear that the simplest of pains is never simple. Pain is an unpleasant experience, not an injury, and it is always affected by many factors. We are beginning to understand the mechanisms by which these other factors can intrude on your perception of injury. It is clear that anxiety, fear, hopelessness, anger, sleeplessness and inactivity all always play their part. This fact does not mean that you are mad but that you are reacting to your situation as a whole human being. This has raised the possibility that psychologists and psychiatrists can help not just crazy people but everyone in pain so that you can act and react in a way which helps.

Dr Peck's book is a fine example from this new school. She writes from her considerable experience with patients in pain. She recruits you to play a part in the treatment team. By doing that, she is not abandoning you to your own devices. A large expanding research effort is in progress to find diagnoses and cure and symptomatic relief. The professionals you see are embarrassed and frustrated by their failures to help you. Those close to you also react in their way to their inability to give successful aid. You are not alone. This book is careful and caring and will help you to place your pain in its surroundings.

Professor Patrick D. Wall, DM, FRCP
Director, Cerebral Functions Research Group
University College London

Preface

Over the last decade clinics devoted specifically to the treatment of chronic pain have been established around the world, and their numbers continue to grow. All this activity stems from a recognition in the medical community of persistent pain as a distinct syndrome, and one that afflicts a vast number of people. Secondly, the growth of Pain Clinics has been greatly encouraged by the development of effective treatment methods for helping sufferers of chronic pain to lead happier, more normal lives. Dr Wilbert Fordyce at the University of Washington Medical School pioneered the work on conditioning chronic pain patients discussed in this book.

Unfortunately, there are still not enough Pain Clinics in the United Kingdom to treat all of those patients with chronic pain. And many of these clinics are not as well funded as their counterparts elsewhere so they do not always have a full range of treatment programmes. For those who wish to consult their doctors about referral to one of the established Pain Clinics, a list of clinics and their addresses is given in the appendix of this book (see page 202).

However, since there are not yet enough Pain Clinics to meet the demand for their services, and also since there are people

1

for whom institutional treatment may not be the best route, this book attempts to make available, on a self-help basis, some of the ideas that have been shown to be useful in the clinical setting. Of course, the book can also serve as an adjunct to therapy in a Pain Clinic. It offers rationales and guidelines that should be useful in either situation. If you intend to use this book solely on a self-help basis, you should consult your doctor before embarking on such a programme to be sure that he agrees with your planned activities and to be sure that this programme is suitable for your type of pain problem.

Finally, the approach to both the problem and the treatment of pain, as outlined in this book, is relatively new. The notions concerning the chronic pain syndrome and the strategies for dealing with it may be as unfamiliar to many doctors as they are to their patients. Therefore, it is hoped that the information which follows will be helpful not only to the people who suffer from chronic pain, but also to medical, paramedical and psychological professionals who care for them.

1. No, You're Not a Hypochondriac

During Roger's last month of work before his retirement from the Navy at age 50, he was hit by a box from a loading crane. He seemed to be all right at the time, but a few days later he was beset by frequent headaches, ringing in the ears, dizziness, and pain and numbness in both his arms and legs. Over the three years after his accident, he had been to many doctors and had tried numerous treatment procedures, but nothing had worked to relieve his symptoms.

Before the accident, Roger not only worked hard but played hard. On weekends, he had enjoyed gardening and playing sports with his five teenagers. Since then, however, he and his life had changed. He now stayed home, doing only some minor cooking, while his wife, an interior decorator, went to work. Gradually he abdicated more and more of his former activities and responsibilities. He gave up boating, driving the car, disciplining the children, making family decisions and managing the family budget.

After one of his doctors hinted to his wife that Roger might be exaggerating his symptoms, she began looking for discrepancies in his behaviour and wondering whether he was sometimes making the most of his pain. Roger was aware of her suspicion, and perhaps because of it, talked about his headaches constantly. He felt angry that he was doubted. The relationship between Roger and his wife, which had previously been good, deteriorated and sexual contact stopped altogether. Each felt frustrated and angry at the other, as well as at the medical professionals who had failed to solve their problems.

When pain becomes a chronic condition, a predictable set of problems are likely to befall those who suffer from it. Some of these problems can, in turn, further aggravate the pain, eventually creating a vicious downward spiral of compounding pain and complex new sets of problems. Such complications can take many forms. The most common involve: trying one unsuccessful treatment after another; losing faith in doctors; taking too many drugs or too much alcohol; worrying about drug dependency; giving up activities from which pleasure and mastery were previously achieved; pain and illness becoming the focus in one's conversation and thoughts; depression; marital discord; feelings of anger, guilt and anxiety; and finally low self-esteem. All of these add up to what will be called the Chronic Pain Trap.

Simply understanding the process as an identifiable syndrome is often comforting to the chronic pain sufferer, since the knowledge helps him to combat the feeling that he is alone with his problem and that no one else understands what is happening to him. Families, doctors and friends sometimes express doubts about the reality of a chronic pain sufferer's experience, implying that they are wondering if, perhaps, the pain is really exaggerated or imagined. Such misunderstanding of the problem only serves to aggravate the condition of the pain sufferer, to make him feel angry with others and eventually to cause him to have negative thoughts about himself. These feelings are, of course, unnecessary and unproductive for everyone concerned.

Chronic pain, as referred to in this book, is pain which has lasted more than a few months, occurs frequently and in some cases continually, and has not responded to appropriate medical treatment. Many readers will have suffered pain for years. In fact, it has been estimated that more than a million Britons suffer from chronic pain. The most common forms involve low back pain, headaches, facial pain and neck or shoulder pain. Abdominal pain, pain in the arms or legs and pain in other localized areas also occur with regularity. Other people find that their pain is more general or spreading.

In some cases chronic pain patients have pain which results from a clearly diagnosable cause, for example arthritis, or nerve damage caused by injury. However, in other situations, the origin of the pain simply cannot be identified. There are in fact three ways to categorize these pain problems:

1 well-defined pain syndromes for which specific treatment procedures are effective;
2 pain problems where the origin of the pain is diagnosed but no satisfactory or lasting treatment procedure exists;
3 pain problems in which neither the cause nor an effective treatment procedure is known.

This book was written for the last two types of problems, where the pain has continued indefinitely, frustrating all attempts to alleviate it. The Chronic Pain Trap and the procedures suggested in this book for reducing the impact of pain on one's life apply equally to pain problems resulting from identifiable or undiagnosed cause. Some sections of the book are addressed more specifically to the patient with pain of undiagnosed origin, since he carries the extra burden of frustration, fear and sometimes suspicion associated with not knowing the cause of his pain.

Experts freely admit that pain is a condition which medical science does not yet completely understand and for which foolproof treatment procedures do not yet exist. The fact that there are so many chronic pain sufferers only serves to demonstrate that this is a type of problem that doctors, in many cases, simply cannot fix up or cure, despite their best efforts.

Indeed, one important aspect of the Chronic Pain Trap is the *expectation* by the patient and his family (and often doctors as well) that medical treatment *can* make the pain go away. In our society, we have so much faith in our medical profession that we firmly believe that it has *all* the answers to our health problems. Pain, however, like the common cold, cancer or heart disease is often beyond the range of current medical understanding.

A patient goes to the doctor expecting to find out what is the cause of the pain and what is the cure. Unfortunately, the doctor may not have either answer. Some physicians will admit this more freely than others. Doctors, after all, are human beings and like to live up to their patients' expectations and be seen as helpful. The doctor who admits he does *not* know the cause of the patient's problem and simply labels it as 'undiagnosed pain' often comes in for harsh criticism. The patient may respond by going off in search of a more 'competent' doctor who hopefully will know the answers. The process of diagnosis and treatment 'shopping' may go on until the patient eventually does find a doctor who suggests a possible cause and is willing to prescribe a treatment procedure. However, if the treatment procedure is not as effective as the patient expects it should be, this doctor does not fare much better. The search is renewed for yet another specialist who will have the *right* answers. This process may go on and on, until doctor after doctor, specialist after specialist has been visited, and operation after operation, medication after medication, treatment after treatment (physiotherapy, acupuncture, manipulation, braces, biofeedback, relaxation therapy and so on) have been tried.

In time, doubts creep in. The specialist and the family, clinging to their belief in medical science, begin to think it is the *patient's* fault that he's not responding to treatment. And they communicate this in subtle or not-so-subtle ways. After all, with the best medical science has to offer and all these doctors and treatments, shouldn't the patient be getting well? Questions are raised concerning whether the patient is malingering, imagining his pain, trying to 'get out of something' or trying to 'get attention'. Words like 'functional' or 'secondary gain' crop up in medical reports. Slowly the suspicion builds. The patient may be watched more closely by the family for any tell-tale discrepancy in his behaviour; while at the same time, the family may feel guilty for having these kinds of doubts. Such suspicion and guilt may, in turn, cause family friction and arguments.

Meanwhile the pain patient is left with the burden of having to prove his innocence. He becomes angry with doctors for not meeting his expectations of being made pain-free, and angrier still that *he* is being blamed for what he perceives as *their* failure. He becomes all the more insistent that he is in pain and that he wants to get well. To prove the point, he goes to more doctors, tries more treatments, feels more and more angry, loses his faith in doctors and becomes more hostile and challenging to medical professionals whom he feels are withholding something from him—freedom from pain.

No physician enjoys dealing with a hostile, angry patient. The normal, human response is to do one of several things. The first may be to send the patient to someone else for care; this may be perceived by the patient as rejection and often leads to even more anger. This is especially likely when the referral is to a psychiatrist or psychologist, which may imply to the patient (although it is often not the case) that he is being considered a 'nut' or a 'hypochondriac'. The second response a doctor may have is to give in to a patient's demands for more medication, more surgery or more of some other form of treatment, whether or not he feels it will do much good. But the continued treatments often are not likely to provide much real relief and can even lead to new complications. Indeed, the 'cure' becomes worse than the disease.

If the patient who is referred for psychological or psychiatric therapy refuses to go, he fears this will confirm his physician's suspicions that he can be 'found out'. Just as people seem to believe in the all-healing power of the medical profession, so they seem to believe in the myth of the 'all seeing' or psychic powers of psychiatrists or psychologists. The patient may go to his appointments, but he is not happy about it. By now he doesn't believe anyone can help him.

Obviously the story doesn't stop there. In fact, it is only the beginning; the rest will be examined in the following chapters. If what you have read so far is starting to sound familiar, you may be someone with chronic pain syndrome, a condition for which there is often no instant medical cure, but you need not despair since there are things you can do which can lead to your living a more normal life in spite of pain. This book will show you ways to cope with your pain.

The first thing to do toward leading a more normal life is to realize that you *are* normal. You are not a hypochondriac; you are not crazy; you are not imagining or exaggerating your pain; you are not weak or undisciplined or anything else. You just have chronic pain syndrome. You are responding in exactly the same way as any other human being (including your doctor, your spouse or your psychologist) would if given the same set of circumstances. One of the first and most basic problems is that you *expect* that you should be able to be made well and pain-free by the medical profession and you have been concentrating all of your efforts on that goal. Your learning (and almost everyone else's) has trained you that if you are sick or in pain, you should go to a doctor to find out what is wrong and to get well—as simple as that. But is it so simple? It would be nice if taking the right pill solved every problem, but as you will come to realize, the answers aren't always so easy. In fact, as we shall discuss in the next chapter, the notion that one takes medication to make oneself well can, and often does, backfire in the case of *chronic* pain.

It may not be easy, but it is important that you now change some long-held beliefs. As long as you keep looking for the instant cure, the cycle, with all its frustrations and disappointments, will continue. Perhaps it is time you said to yourself: 'I have done all the treatment-shopping any normal person can be expected to do. It's time to give up working on finding the instant cure. It's not my fault that I still have pain, and it's not my doctor's fault either. Medical science just doesn't completely understand pain yet. But if there's a way to learn to cope better with chronic pain, I'm ready to try it.' If you are at the point where you can say this to yourself, read on. You are the person this book is addressing. If you are not yet ready to accept that you may have to find ways to 'live with' your pain and are still seeking an 'instant cure', perhaps you are not far enough into the story of chronic pain. When you are ready though, the procedures described here will still work and you come back and try them then.

It should be clear by now that you cannot be a hypochondriac if so many people with the same or similar problems are responding in exactly the same way. And the evidence now massively supports that fact. The problem is not with *you*. It is with your beliefs and expectations about the medical system. Changing your expectations can make a big difference. Accepting yourself as *normal* can make a big difference. Being accepted as normal by your family and doctor can make a big difference. Eventually, you may wish to have them read this book as well, since surprisingly few people understand these simple facts. Being accepted as normal will not, however, solve your problems all by itself. But it may make you feel a little better and a little more like trying again, and that is an important prerequisite to following the rest of the self-help programme outlined in this book. Accepting yourself as normal can reduce your anxiety about being considered a hypochondriac by others, and may reduce the feeling that you need to keep proving your pain by going to new doctors and trying new treatment procedures. You are not a hypochondriac. You are perfectly normal!

2. The Chronic Pain Trap

The set of problems connected with the chronic pain syndrome is fairly complex. Therefore, it is important to consider each of its aspects in some detail. The general downward spiral of problems can be referred to as the Chronic Pain Trap. But the Chronic Pain Trap is, in fact, composed of a number of more specific and definable traps. Of course not all chronic pain sufferers have encountered all of the traps listed below, but more than likely you will find that some apply to you.

The Medication Trap

George, aged 37, was a primary school teacher until he injured his back a few years ago in a fall down a staircase. Since standing aggravated his pain, he was advised to give up his teaching. After two back surgeries, neither of which relieved his pain, his doctor prescribed codeine and advised him to rest. Over a six year period, the frequency and amount of the codeine gradually increased until George was taking enormous amounts every day; yet he was still not receiving sufficient pain relief. When the Drug Investigatory Committee of his state set up guidelines for drug ceilings, the doctor suddenly reduced the codeine prescription by half. George had been taking *twice* the amount recommended as a *ceiling* by the Committee.

This sudden severe reduction caused George to become very agitated. He called his senator to complain about his doctor and then found another doctor who would give him more codeine. Finally, in desperation, George's doctor referred him to a Pain Clinic. George was caught in the Medication Trap.

Next to our faith in doctors is our faith in the powers of medication. Most of us believe that when we are sick or in pain, a little of the right kind of medicine is all that's needed to fix us up. To prove our faith, we take millions of dollars worth of pain killers every year. And for short term problems, such as pulled muscles, the occasional headache or pain following surgery, analgesics work fine. For this type of temporary ailment, they are effective. However, when analgesics are used on a continual basis they can lead to an unfortunate new problem — the Medication Trap.

One important aspect of the Medication Trap has to do with what is called *tolerance*. Tolerance is the body's gradual adjustment to drugs. Our bodies have a built-in mechanism which adjusts to the presence of drugs in our systems and causes us to gradually require more and more of the given drug in order to get the same pain-killing effect. Tolerance is built up against all drugs over time, and so no matter which you use, you end up having to take more and more of it to get the same effect.

Obviously this can cause several further problems. One major one is drug dependence. Drug dependence is a frightening term, but unfortunately it denotes a very common problem in the chronic pain syndrome. In the chronic pain context, dependence is not something one chooses to do or something one needs to feel guilty about. It is plainly and simply the inevitable outcome of chronic use of pain killing medication with addictive properties. Many patients never even know that the medication they are taking is potentially addictive; others know about the dangers but think that so long as they are disciplined enough, they can resist dependence.

There are two forms of drug dependence. *Physical de-*

pendence is the sort usually associated with medication containing narcotics and which results in a range of physical withdrawal symptoms when a patient abruptly stops taking the medication. *Psychological dependence* refers to the habit of taking drugs, but a habit that is so ingrained that withdrawal of the drug causes symptoms of psychological stress. Most chronic pain sufferers do not believe that they are subject to either of these types of dependence but, in fact, those who have taken pain killers for a long time will suffer from one or both, depending on the types of medication they use. It is not important, however, to establish whether you are psychologically or physically dependent on drugs. The main point is that if you have been taking pain killers for a long time, you are by now probably taking far too many for your body's health (drugs are very hard on your kidneys and liver) and getting far too little relief (if any) from them. All drugs (even the caffeine in your coffee) are toxic or poisonous in large enough doses. Many patients are told by their doctors that they must stop their gradually increasing dose of analgesics when they reach a given dosage, since to increase the intake further would be approaching a toxic level. However, because a patient's body has been slowly building up a tolerance to the drug, he may be getting little or no benefit from even massive amounts of pain killer. Unfortunately, patients are not always told or do not always understand this tolerance-toxicity problem. They often assume that if a little doesn't work, more will and that the sky is the limit. Nothing could be more incorrect.

Most pain patients feel guilty about taking drugs. They worry about what their doctor, friends or family will think. Yet they remain ambivalent about drugs because they still hold to the belief that medication *will* help. After all, they've had years of past experience with drug-produced relief for short-term pain problems; moreover, drugs may have been initially effective for their now chronic pain problem. And all forms of the media constantly push medication as the answer to problems. Thus, chronic pain patients find themselves continuing to want to try various medications or asking for more and more analgesics, but all the while feeling more guilty about their increasing intake.

This ambivalence leads to some curious behaviour. Just as the overweight person may occasionally but unwisely try to lose weight by starvation diets, the chronic pain sufferer (or his doctor) may, from time to time, decide he is taking too much medication and try to cut back. If the cut-back is too rapid or in some other way is not done correctly, it can prove to be an aversive experience for both patient and doctor, as well as being almost as impossible to maintain as the starvation diet. Such a trial often results in the onset of a particularly bad attack of pain which in turn leads to the need for as much or more medication than had previously been prescribed. Such an outcome is self-defeating and strengthens fears in both the patient and the doctor that the patient is drug dependent.

Another behaviour which may emerge occurs when a patient obtains prescriptions for pain-killers from more than one doctor without informing the other doctor(s) involved. Initially, patients keep their secret out of a sense of guilt; later this is complicated by the fear of being cut off. However, this practice can become very dangerous, not only because of the risks of toxicity, but also because some mixtures of different drugs can result in unexpected, compound effects. The layman is rarely sophisticated enough to understand the hazards.

Patients often find themselves taking medication in private to avoid comment from family or friends. This, among other things, may lead to irregular patterns of drug intake. Thus, chronic medication users may not be aware of how much they take or when they last took medication. This may be particularly true when a pain episode is severe and a patient has already taken a fair amount of medication, causing him to be somewhat less alert than usual. It is no wonder that chronic pain patients have, on occasion, accidentally overdosed.

Joan, a 20 year-old with chronic headaches of six years' duration, had lived with and kept house for her elderly grandfather since her completion of high school. When one doctor failed to relieve her headaches, she went to another and then another. Each doctor prescribed new medications and Joan tried them all. Then, whenever she had a really bad headache, Joan would go to her medicine cabinet and begin taking pills until the headache finally went away. After her boyfriend found her unconscious on a couple of occasions, she was referred to a Pain Clinic for treatment. When, at the request of the Pain Clinic, Joan agreed to having her boyfriend clean out the medicine cabinet, he brought in a grocery bag, filled with over a hundred bottles of pills. Joan was caught in the Medication Trap.

Another notable aspect of the Medication Trap is the fact that medication may actually help to maintain high levels of pain. This is a complex process which is difficult to explain, but the critical factor is *timing*. Patients often wait until their pain has become severe before taking a pill or an injection. The medicine then yields a pleasant sensation of temporary relief. Since relief is a positive sensation, it has a way, if repeated often enough, of actually reinforcing not only medicine-taking but also the pain which preceded it. Psychologists have identified a law of behaviour that says that removal of something aversive strengthens the behaviour which precedes it. In this case, pain and medication-taking precede relief and actually may be strengthened by the conditioning pattern which occurs.

Thus, pain medication taken on a chronic or permanent basis loses its effectiveness and may even serve to maintain or increase the problem. In addition, tolerance leads to larger doses which, besides being worrisome and guilt-producing, produce even more dangerous health risks. It can cause you, your family and your doctor needless worry and conflict, not to mention deteriorating physical health.

Does the Medication Trap sound like one in which you may be caught? Chapter 7 will explain a fairly painless way to gradually work out of this trap.

The Take It Easy Trap

Ann, a 39 year-old housewife and mother, suffered chronic back pain due to a malformation of her spine. As a younger woman she had been very active, doing all the housework and cooking for her family, being co-leader of the Girl Guides and taking piano lessons and bookkeeping classes. She enjoyed shopping, visiting neighbours and family outings. However the back pain she experienced when lifting her children led her to the doctor, who advised her to 'take it easy'. Taking this advice seriously, she had, over the years, gradually given up activities until she was reduced to doing nothing but a little dusting, preparing menus and knitting. She did not feel that she could ride in a car for more than ten minutes, and this further reduced such outside activities as shopping. The oldest daughter took over all the housekeeping activities, with Ann taking a supervisory role, saying that if only she could do them, she would be able to do them so much better. Ann had to be dressed and put into her back brace by her daughter. A neighbour did her shopping and washed her hair. She was afraid to climb the stairs in their two-storey house for fear of hurting her back, so she crawled up and down. She also avoided lifting or pushing against anything over half a kilo, so her family had to open doors for her, hold the telephone receiver, and perform all sorts of small errands. From time to time she would try to cook, but her daughter had to lift the pans, open the oven and cupboard doors, stir thick consistencies and so on. Ann and her family were caught in the Take It Easy Trap.

Chronic pain sufferers frequently say that certain physical exertions aggravate pain. Doctors often advise patients to take it easy or prescribe bed rest. Following this advice, patients may quit their jobs and go into retirement. At home, families take over the household chores and scold the chronic pain sufferer who tries to take on any work around the house. One of the problems with taking it easy, however, is that activities that were once enjoyed begin to drop away along with those which were aversive or difficult. Along with mowing the lawn or vacuuming the carpet, favourite sports may be ruled out, holidays and outings become difficult and less frequent. Friends initially make special considerations and are sympathetic, but in time they fade away as well. No one likes to have friends who can't do things and who have nothing left to talk about except pain.

This becomes a trap at several levels. First, when one is inactive, muscles very quickly become weak. They may become so weak that pain is aggravated by any sudden or unusual physical exertion. Thus, a sudden urge to mow the lawn or wash the car may result in severe muscle strain. Patients and families quickly learn that particularly bad pain attacks may follow such exertions and any further similar urges are discouraged or even punished. But this means muscles only become weaker and weaker and more and more activities become too difficult to do.

An even more insidious problem is the depression which accompanies massive loss of activities, pleasure, friends, work, and other interests. In a society such as ours in which the work ethic is so important, loss of work (including housework) can have profound effects on mood, motivation, thinking, and self-image. One begins to see oneself as weak, unable to provide, and generally not pulling one's own weight.

There is a great deal of discussion about whether getting to take time off from work and receive temporary or permanent compensation might be a reason that some patients have chronic pain, either consciously or unconsciously. Perhaps this is the case with a few people, but clinical experience indicates that it is the exception rather than the rule. The punishment that results from not working in a society such as ours far outweighs the reward. There may be some initial rewards for people who retreat from work, but the punishing consequences usually catch up before long and depression sets in, especially since many pleasurable activities are usually lost in the process.

Plans and dreams are abandoned as they are considered no longer possible. Goals and things to look forward to disappear. In short, all of those things which people need to maintain normal good mental health are lost and the patient becomes more and more depressed. For these reasons depression and chronic pain often go hand in hand. As will be seen in a later section, depression, too, can serve to aggravate pain while loss of activity fuels the depression, creating a vicious cycle.

Finally, *time* becomes a problem for the chronic pain sufferer. If you can't be active, there just aren't many things that you can do to fill your time. The days become long and tedious.

The Depression Trap

Maria, a 45 year-old housewife and mother of two teenagers, suffered low back pain after lifting a heavy load at the meat packing factory where she worked. After several operations, physiotherapy, and acupuncture, her pain was worse than ever. She spent most of her day in a dressing gown, doing little but watching television and resting. She cried frequently. Maria felt that her husband was unsympathetic and she suspected him of having an affair. Her children were busy being teenagers and didn't have much time for her. She felt lonely, depressed, unloved, unappreciated and good-for-nothing. One Saturday, when she and her husband had planned to go to the races together, Maria said at the last minute she felt too bad to go. When her husband went on without her, she took an overdose of her pain medication. Fortunately, one of her children found her unconscious in time to call the ambulance and save her life. Maria was caught in the Depression Trap.

The onset of depression which accompanies inactivity brings on yet another host of problems which further adds to the burden of the chronic pain sufferer. Feelings of worthlessness and despair frequently accompany depression. Motivation and the desire to do activities previously enjoyed are much reduced. Things lose their pleasantness and the whole range of activities which previously seemed exciting begins to seem dull and uninteresting. Even the slightest effort appears to be an impossible task so that eventually the patient doubts his own ability to do *anything*—even things easily accomplished in the past. The patient may find himself feeling blue or having unexplained fits of crying or moping. Sleep becomes disturbed. He has trouble falling asleep or awakens early and can't get back to sleep. This, in turn, may lead to a reliance on sleep

17

medication which has all of the same difficulties discussed in the section on the Medication Trap. In addition, depression has been found to increase the perception or feeling of pain. Research has shown that after the very same painful procedures (such as the same type of surgery), patients who are depressed report more pain than those who are not depressed. Thus, while it is a natural outcome of the hopeless feelings which accompany continual treatment failures, the withdrawal of normal activities and the unrelenting pain itself, depression also aggravates the pain problem.

Some people think the pain sufferer has it made and that a life of retirement would be terrific. Sure, reading and watching television are fun, but day after day it becomes tedious, and the accompanying problems are anything but fun.

The Complaint-Resentment-Guilt Trap

Glenda, a 42 year-old woman, married to a doctor had suffered low back pain for four years. After repeated attempts at various types of treatment from the best surgeons and doctors in the country, Glenda still suffered pain. Even the large amount of medication seemed to give her little relief. Fearing that she would aggravate the pain by even mild effort, Glenda became increasingly inactive. She gave up the part-time nursing job that she had resumed when her daughter had reached school age. The active social life that Glenda and her husband had once enjoyed dropped away to nothing as invitations had to be repeatedly turned down. Entertaining at home became all but impossible.

Glenda found that pain had come to dominate her life. It was difficult to think about anything else at all. She tried not to talk about it, but her husband, Don, could tell by her facial expressions that she was in pain and he often asked how she was feeling. Don tried hard to be understanding. He tried to cut back his busy practice so that he could spend more time with Glenda and their daughter. They hired a housekeeper.

From time to time, however, Glenda and Don had loud arguments in which they accused each other of not understanding the burden each of them carried. These fights usually ended with

Don storming out of the house to cool off, leaving Glenda in tears. A few minutes later, they would make up and retract all the accusations they had hurled at each other. Neither of them could explain how the arguments started, and both felt at a loss to account for the increasing bitterness displayed during these outbursts. Yet they went on, becoming worse and worse. Glenda and Don were caught in the Complaint-Resentment-Guilt Trap.

When the chronic pain sufferer has ceased normal activities, both because those activities could aggravate pain and because they are now punished by others, the number of topics of conversation the patient has to talk about becomes greatly reduced. In addition, between the lethargy introduced by depression and the normal irritability caused by pain, the chronic pain sufferer is not an easy person to live with. By now his problem has become the main focus of his life and therefore of nearly all of his conversation and action.

Most chronic pain patients say that they try very hard not to complain to the family, but when you look carefully at their conversation or actions, much of it is related to their problem. A chronic pain sufferer may not tell his family *directly* that he is in pain but family members usually know by the fact that the patient is resting, taking medication, has a drawn expression, has trouble getting out of chairs, rubs his back or head, limps, winces, moves slowly and carefully, talks about his doctor or latest treatment, or is just generally grouchy. There is more than one way to complain.

These kinds of complaints are perfectly normal and it is not something chronic pain sufferers need to feel guilty about. It simply needs to be understood that this and the associated problems of chronic pain also have a profound effect on the family. All human relationships are based on reciprocity. Couple interaction studies have shown that couples who are doing well together are giving each other fairly equal amounts of positive and/or negative feedback. In other words, couples who are getting along give each other approximately equal amounts of positive attention (hugs, kisses, loving words, sex, special considerations) and approximately equal amount of negative attention (bitchiness, grouchiness, argumentative-ness, angry retorts, accusations, ignoring, silent treatment). It is when this reciprocity breaks down and one partner feels he is having to give more than he gets in return that troubles begin.

Such a situation often becomes a reality for the chronic pain patient, whose condition puts a much greater burden on all family members, who have to assume the patient's share of household duties and whose activities are curtailed by a family member who can't go along on outings or does so but has to have special consideration. The chronic pain sufferer's needs are often put above other family members' needs. Loyal and loving family members can tolerate this situation for a short period of time, but due to the continuing lack of reciprocity, the normal human responses of anger and resentment eventually catch up with them. Since the chronic pain patient *is* loved by the family, guilt accompanies the anger and resentment. What we see developing then, is an interaction pattern characterized by anger and guilt. The family or partner becomes resentful and in some way blows off steam at the chronic pain patient, but once he has rid himself of his angry emotions, he starts considering what a tough time the patient really must be having. He begins feeling guilty and solicitous. On the other hand, the pain patient feels angry that the partner doesn't understand, and he is resentful that the 'well' partner has all the things the pain patient is missing—good health, activities and friends. The pain patient then lets off steam or becomes resentful in return. Once this pressure is released, the patient reconsiders and realizes how kind and considerate the partner has really been and in turn he feels guilty and solicitous toward the partner. This interplay of feelings between pain patients and their partners or family eventually becomes the dominant theme of the relationship. The family interaction becomes defined by this resentment-guilt cycle. At the same time, this breakdown in healthy family relations is often denied or just not recognized. All of our learning leads us to believe that it is shameful to express anger or resentment toward someone who is sick.

How this resentment-guilt interaction is played out differs according to a family's or couple's fighting style. Some couples have fairly direct arguments, openly accusing one another of playing the pain for all it's worth, or failing to be understanding or sympathetic. Others harbour a more silent resentment which comes out indirectly in more subtle, disguised ways (sarcastic remarks, sympathetic-like behaviour which does not seem genuine, the silent treatment, or preoccupation with other things). These sorts of behaviours, however, do not disguise the underlying tension. Trust and open communication cannot continue to survive in such an environment.

A third variation is possible with couples in which one partner expresses anger more directly than the other. Both partners may be equally hostile, but whereas one expresses hostility openly, the other expresses it through less obvious means. This pattern ia a fairly common one. What is interesting in this variation is that outsiders often side with and feel sympathy for the person who expresses his anger more indirectly, since more subtly-expressed hostility cannot be as readily perceived by those who are not the target. This taking of sides by others often tends to reinforce the pattern—making the overtly angry person (often the pain patient) feel even more angry and misunderstood as he is labelled the villain, while the indirectly angry person becomes more smug, self-righteous and unaware of his own resentment and the transmission of this disguised anger to his partner.

You may be saying to yourself that this sort of interaction pattern doesn't fit your situation. And it is possible that it doesn't; but if you take a serious look at your own interactions with your family, you will probably find some reciprocal resentments. This is a normal response that typically occurs in families in which one family member is chronically disabled, regardless of the type of chronic illness, whether it be heart disease, cancer, stroke or chronic pain. This natural response again violates the notion that we have been taught concerning how we ought to respond to sick people (or from the pain patient's view, how we ought to respond to those who sacrifice to care for us). However, despite our best efforts, disruption of reciprocity usually takes over, resulting in this type of resentment. No matter what we are taught about selfishness, we are basically selfish beings, and if our needs are not met for a long enough time, we react by harbouring resentment. This is an especially uncomfortable feeling precisely because it does violate our teaching. We consider such emotions unacceptable, and facing them causes us discomfort and anxiety. Therefore we are prone to overlook or deny them. You may find, if you are honest with yourself, that you have done exactly that. Due to the discomfort of recognizing these feelings in yourself, you have never confronted them. It should be remembered, though, that denial is a natural response to this situation. It is the rule, not the exception.

Nonetheless, this kind of resentful interaction causes not only emotional strain but physical tension as well, and muscle tension only further aggravates pain. Additionally, this kind of interaction pattern takes the place of more positive reciprocal interactions that may have existed previously. As this happens, the joy disappears from the relationship and the partners may begin to feel that they are held together only by a sense of obligation—after all you can't leave a sick person. Finally, if carried far enough, this becomes the focus of the interaction—the patient, always worried that the partner may leave, binds him by guilt; the partner, effectively bound by this guilt, acts from a sense of obligation. This is, however, only the extreme case in fairly advanced cases of family breakdown.

Of course not all chronic pain patients are married or have families. But it is true that most people have someone who is important in their life—it may be a parent, a child, or a friend. If you do not have a spouse or family, please substitute the word for the important person in your life in the above discussion. Human interaction patterns tend to be similar between people who are close to one another, regardless of the nature of their relationship.

22

Summary

Each section of this chapter shows how the various pitfalls of the Chronic Pain Trap work to compound the pain patient's problems. Many of these are a reaction to the chronic nature of the pain itself or to the continued use of treatment designed for short-term pain problems.

The first step towards resolving the problems of the Chronic Pain Trap is to gain an awareness of one's own special situation. The next chapter will help you assess exactly how you may be ensnared. Subsequent chapters will provide specific suggestions for overcoming each of these traps.

3. Analysing What Chronic Pain Has Done to Your Life

Understanding what chronic pain has done to your life is a difficult task and one that you may find you cannot face easily. It is, nonetheless, an important task since it is the necessary starting point for change. To pick up the threads of life and begin weaving them back into a fabric, it is important to first assess the extent of the damage. Depending on how long you have had chronic pain, this may be easier or more difficult but, in any case, it will involve careful observation and recording of your behaviour. This book will ask you to do a fair amount of record-keeping, make written contracts with yourself, draw up lists, and more. It has been found that this sort of written work is very important to a successful programme and you are encouraged to follow the suggestions rigorously.

Since chronic pain affects the whole family, it is also suggested that you choose someone close to you as a partner who will also read this book and who will from time to time sit down and participate in exercises with you. It can be very helpful to have someone else's view of your problems to contrast and compare with your own, and it also can be advantageous to have someone else's memory, ideas, and suggestions working together with yours at such things as making lists of potential activities, recalling activities in which you used to engage before chronic pain, and so forth. The best person to choose is the one who is most important to you. If you are married a spouse is probably the best choice, even if you now feel that your spouse is unsympathetic. Reading this book and participating in this programme with you should lead your spouse to a greater understanding and a sense of unity with you. A good friend, a parent, or an older child may also be able to participate in this way if you don't have a spouse.

Assessing what chronic pain has done to your life will require honesty—brutal honesty, perhaps—for both you and your partner. As discussed above, it is almost impossible to get out of the Chronic Pain Trap by yourself. If you are serious about following the plan set forth in the following chapters, now is the time to ask your partner to begin reading, either with you or separately, the first two chapters of this book. To be most helpful, and most honest, your partner needs the basic information that we've been discussing.

Once you have both read to this point, each of you will be ready to fill out the **Extent of the Damages Worksheets** on pages 26-8. Each sheet should be filled out *independently* and honestly, and only after careful reading of Chapters 1 and 2. Once you have completely filled them out, they should be shared and discussed in some detail.

It will be important in this discussion not to fall into the Complaint-Resentment-Guilt Trap and end up simply arguing. At the same time, it is essential to share honestly each of your opinions about the nature of the problem. Some of the questions on the worksheet may seem very emotionally charged, but provided you have read Chapters 1 and 2 carefully and have understood and absorbed the information there, you will realize that the various traps described are the natural, normal outcome of your chronic pain syndrome and that you should not feel guilty or defensive about them. What is needed now is not blaming or fault-finding, but a realistic assessment of the extent of the damages so that the targets for change can best be pinpointed. Absolute honesty is needed in order to do this since if *either* of you considers something a problem, some sort of work undoubtedly needs to be done with regard to it.

Since it is important to get your joint efforts with your partner on your chronic pain problem off to a good start, a few rules are listed for joint work:

1. Whenever you and your partner work on a joint exercise, it must be taken as a serious effort. Casual attempts are unlikely to be of much help.

2. During a joint exercise, you and your partner should work away from the distractions of children, television, telephone calls, etc. It is important that you set up times which will minimize these distractions. Both partners should devote full concentration to the task without fear of interruption.

3. These are to be *constructive* sessions and under no circumstances should they be allowed to degenerate into blaming and argumentation. If you find yourself slipping into an argument, stop immediately, do your best to make up and then go back to the target task.

4. Never discuss things other than the target task during these times.

Now you and your partner can sit down and fill out the **Extent of the Damages Worksheets.** Once you have filled them out independently and discussed your answers constructively, you can then go through the reading list on page 29 and mark off the chapters which you need to read. If *either* you or your partner made a mark by any question relevant to a chapter, that chapter should be read by *both* of you.

Extent of the Damages Worksheet —Patient

Place a tick in the box opposite statements you feel are true for your situation.

☐ 1. My doctors sometimes act as if they think that I'm a hypochondriac or that I'm imagining or exaggerating my pain.

☐   2.   My family sometimes acts as if they think that I'm a hypochondriac or that I'm imagining or exaggerating my pain.

☐   3.   I sometimes wonder whether I might really be a hypochondriac, or whether my pain could actually be imagined or exaggerated.

☐   4.   I feel angry when my doctors act as if I'm a hypochondriac.

☐   5.   I feel angry when my family acts as if I'm a hypochondriac.

☐   6.   I feel as if no one understands my predicament.

☐   7.   I have tried many unsuccessful treatments and I am losing my faith in the medical profession.

☐   8.   I sometimes feel angry with my doctors for not being able to cure my pain.

☐   9.   I am worried that I may be caught in the Medication Trap: that is, I feel that I take too much medication or alcohol and get too little relief, but I am reluctant or fearful of stopping.

☐   10.   I feel I may be caught in the Take It Easy Trap: that is, I no longer engage in many activities that I used to enjoy and I feel that this may be affecting my mood and my outlook on life.

☐   11.   I feel I may be caught in the Depression Trap: that is, I have lost motivation, sometimes feel weepy or depressed, lack the energy and drive I used to have, and feel hopeless and despondent.

☐   12.   I feel I may be caught in the Complaint-Resentment-Guilt Trap: that is, I sometimes resent my partner for not understanding when things are all fine for him/her, but then I often feel guilty when I remember how good he/she is to me and what a burden my problem causes to the family.

☐   13.   I feel that my partner may be caught in the Complaint-Resentment-Guilt Trap. I think he/she sometimes resents my pain, my inability to do my share and the burden these things place on the family. However, he/she may feel

27

guilty for this as well, since I know at other times he/she feels sorry for me.

☐ 14. I sometimes feel negative about myself for not being able to cope with pain and not being able to pull my weight in the family.

☐ 15. I feel that there are currently other problems in my life in addition to those mentioned above (such as marital relationship or sexual problems).

Specify: _____

_____

_____

_____

Extent of the Damages Worksheet —Partner

Place a tick in the box opposite statements you feel are true for you and your chronic pain partner's situation.

☐ 1. The doctors sometimes act as if they think my partner is a hypochondriac or is imagining or exaggerating pain.

☐ 2. I sometimes wonder whether my partner is a hypochondriac or is imagining or exaggerating pain.

☐ 3. I feel angry when the doctors act as if my partner might be a hypochondriac.

☐ 4. I feel that I do not fully understand my partner's situation.

☐ 5. I am losing my faith in the medical profession.

☐ 6. I sometimes feel angry at the doctors for not being able to cure my partner's pain.

☐ 7. I think my partner is caught in the Medication Trap: that is, I feel he/she takes too much medication and/or alcohol and gets too little relief but is reluctant or fearful of stopping.

☐   8.   I feel my partner is caught in the Take It Easy Trap: that is, perhaps his/her retirement from meaningful activities is adding to the problem.

☐   9.   I feel my partner may be caught in the Depression Trap: that is, he/she seems to have lost motivation, sometimes is depressed or weepy, lacks the energy and drive he/she used to have, and feels hopeless and despondent.

☐   10.   I feel I am caught in the Complaint-Resentment-Guilt Trap: that is, I sometimes find myself feeling resentful of his/her pain problem and the hardship it imposes on the family, but I often feel guilty for feeling this way, since he/she can't help it.

☐   11.   I feel that my partner may be caught in the Complaint-Resentment-Guilt Trap: that is, he/she often acts as if he/she resents my good health and accuses me of not understanding what it's like to have pain. However, I think he/she also feels guilt at this anger since he/she knows I try hard to take care of him/her to the best of my ability.

☐   12.   I feel that there are currently other problems in my life in addition to those mentioned above (such as marital relationship or sexual problems).

Specify: _____

_____

_____

_____

Reading List

You and your partner should now go over your **Extent of the Damages Worksheets**. If either of you have ticked any statements, both of you should read the relevant chapter listed below. Mark the chapters you need to read and refer back to this page as a guide.

Controlling Chronic Pain

Patient's Worksheet	Partner's Worksheet	Chapter to Read
1, 4, 6, 7, 8, 9	1, 3, 5, 6, 7	4. Your Doctor and You
10, 11, 14	8, 9	5. How to Resume More Normal Activity
3, 11, 14	9	6. Fighting Off the Depression of Chronic Pain
9	7	7. Controlling the Pain Killers
Reading for all patients	Reading for all partners	8. What to Do and What Not to Do When You Are in Pain
Reading for all patients	Reading for all partners	9. How You, the Family, Can Help
Reading for all patients		10. Preventing Pain
12, 13, 15	10, 11, 12	11. Recognizing and Solving Other Problems Which May Aggravate Pain
Reading for all patients		12. Maintaining Your Progress

Before you go on to read those chapters, you need to set about collecting more information on yourself. This will be an important step, as it will tell you exactly where to begin your self-help programme, and it will give you additional feedback concerning the specific areas which will be tackled in later chapters as they apply to you.

Information Collecting on Current Activity: The Activity Diary

You should now start keeping an **Activity Diary** each day for
30

Example Activity Diary

Time	Activity
7.15	Breakfast made for family
8.00	Returned to bed to rest
10.30	Made coffee and read newspaper
10.55	Did half the breakfast dishes
11.10	Watched news on television
11.30	Watched television
12.05	Made a sandwich for lunch
12.30	Finished breakfast dishes
12.55	Talked with friend on phone
1.20	Rested on couch and knitted
2.30	Ironed two shirts
3.00	Rested in bed
3.30	Children home from school, prepared snack
4.00	Started dinner
4.30	Watched television with children
5.00	Finished dinner preparations
6.15	Ate dinner with family
7.00	Watched television
8.30	Had hot bath
9.00	Watched television
10.10	Went to bed

Controlling Chronic Pain

Activity Diary

Time	Activity

the next three to five days. Exactly how long you keep the diary is up to you. The main idea is to collect enough information to form a truly representative picture of the way you spend your time. The outline for keeping this type of diary is shown on pages 31-2. The **Activity Diary** will show you how you divide your time between activities, including resting; and it will help you plan the times at which you could fit in new activities.

Your **Activity Diary** should always be kept handy so that it can be filled out as the day goes by. This ensures that you don't miss anything. If you go out of the house, it can be carried along in a purse or pocket. It only takes a few seconds to take it out and jot down your latest activity. If you find it really impossible to fill out as you go during the day (as a few people seem to), then sit down at lunch, at dinner, and just before going to bed and catch up on your record of the previous portion of the day's activities. It is, however, crucial that you work on the diary at least three times a day to assure its accuracy. You may want to show it to your partner after making an entry to make sure you haven't forgotten anything which he or she might remember.

Information Collecting on Potential Activities

The task for the next exercise will be to make a very long list of all sorts of activities which you either used to do before your pain problem or that you have never done but would like to do. The list should be·at *least* thirty activities long; fifty is better. An example of this list is shown on pages 34-5. It is good to work with your partner on this because people often have difficulty doing it alone. Many of the activities on your list will be things which you cannot do at the moment and which you may feel you will never be able to do again. But don't worry about that at this point. Write everything down. Making this list may take a lot of effort, but it will be well worth the work. If you stop short of thirty activities, you both need to keep working until you reach that minimum goal.

Example Potential Activities

1.	Window shopping
2.	Shopping for new clothes
3.	Swimming
4.	Going to a movie
5.	Cleaning cupboard
6.	Ironing
7.	Using sewing machine
8.	Visiting my relatives interstate
9.	Going out to dinner at a restaurant
10.	Taking a course at night
11.	Shopping for groceries by myself
12.	Going on a picnic with the family
13.	Going to a drive-in movie
14.	Camping in our caravan
15.	Cleaning the back porch
16.	Going to the hairdressers
17.	Weeding the garden
18.	Planting a flower bed
19.	Having friends over for dinner

20.	Driving Mary to piano lessons
21.	Throwing a party
22.	Having lunch with a friend
23.	Golfing
24.	Going to the races
25.	Watercolour painting
26.	Volunteer work at Cancer Society
27.	Attending a parent-teacher's meeting
28.	Planning a romantic weekend
29.	Making new curtains for the kitchen
30.	Learning to play the guitar

Potential Activities

1.	
2.	
3.	
4.	
5.	
6.	
7.	

8.	
9.	
10.	
11.	
12.	
13.	
14.	
15.	
16.	
17.	
18.	
19.	
20.	
21.	
22.	
23.	
24.	
25.	
26.	
27.	

28.	
29.	
30.	

Information Collecting on How You Complain

It is also helpful to know exactly how you express your pain to the world. Everybody talks about how they feel. But there are other ways of expressing pain or pleasure, comfort or discomfort, than with words: they are referred to as nonverbal communication. Especially in close relationships, we become very skilled at reading each other's nonverbal as well as verbal behaviour. At the same time, we don't often stop to think about or analyse our habits for nonverbal expression. It is good to know what you are doing that tells others you are in pain, and you can grasp it if you take time to notice.

This exercise can be accomplished by observing yourself carefully over a similar three to five days of information collecting. Each time you notice you are expressing pain, note it down on a 'complaint list' divided into verbal or nonverbal categories. You may want to ask your partner to keep a list too. At the end of the observation period, you can compare notes. This should be an interesting exercise rather than a threatening, accusing or defensive one. The main purpose is to increase your awareness so that you can go on to follow the self-help suggestions outlined in Chapters 8 and 9. If you think about it, chances are you will find that you show pain in ways you did not realize.

Summary

Now that you have collected information concerning your current activity, your potential activity and your complaint behaviour, you are ready to begin plans for your self-help programme. It is suggested that you read the next four chapters thoroughly and then check with your doctor before actually starting. It is wise to consult your doctor first since there may be a *few* cases in which activities that form a part of your plan should be eliminated or the medication aspect of the programme should not be followed for medical reasons. If you are one of these cases you should know it and act according to medical advice. Your doctor will probably agree that cutting down on your medication is a good idea and that *gradual* and *systematic* building of activities (as will be suggested in the next chapter) is a good idea. It may be helpful to have your doctor read this book as well, so that he/she will be aware of the rationale for these suggestions.

4. Your Doctor and You

Doctor-patient relationships are often very special ones. In our culture and most others, doctors hold an honoured place as those entrusted with the special knowledge to be able to cure sickness or at least ease symptoms (such as pain). As advisors to personal health, they also serve a general function as confidants for their patients. Thus, patients look up to their doctors, whom they see as masters of the art of medicine.

Both doctor and patient have specific and well-defined roles in the usual doctor-patient relationship. The patient's role is to seek all possible help, report honestly all complaints, and to follow doctor's orders. The doctor's role is to diagnose the malady correctly, prescribe the right treatment, explain the illness and the treatment to the patient and give the patient some indication of the time needed for the cure. In most cases, this conventional doctor-patient relationship works well. Many problems can be clearly diagnosed and the treatment of choice prescribed with reasonably predictable results. Thus, usually doctor and patient are reinforced in their respective roles as helper and seeker of help.

With chronic pain, however, the usual doctor-patient roles often do not work as well, or fail altogether. The reason for this is that there simply may not *be* a medical solution to *your* pain problem, at least at this time. Medicine, although it has overcome many barriers in recent years, is still unable to solve many problems or illnesses and chronic pain, except for the few known pain syndromes, is one of these. That is, in fact, what chronic pain means: pain problems which haven't been solved. You may wish to refer back to Chapter 1, 'No, You're Not a Hypochondriac', where this notion is explained more fully.

Since patients continue to *expect* the doctor to be able to solve any problem, including chronic pain, he or she is placed in a very difficult position. Patients continue to come for help and solutions, and the doctor generally continues to try to satisfy these demands. But, as one 'solution' after another fails, both patient and doctor become more frustrated. 'Solutions' may involve being sent to a specialist, physiotherapy, acupuncture, manipulation, medication, braces, traction, biofeedback, or surgery—sometimes multiple operations. You may have tried other 'solutions' that you can add to the list.

As these 'solutions' continue to fail, the patient often loses faith in the doctor. At the same time the doctor loses faith in his client, deciding that this patient must *want* to have pain or be sick. At this point, the special doctor-patient relationship begins to break down. And as this happens, the patient often begins to feel rejected. This can lead to a frenzied attempt on the patient's part to more vehemently *demand* attention and help. Some patients end up pestering their doctors, calling them frequently to explain their latest symptoms, asking for more and more medication, insisting on surgery, or sometimes just generally hounding them for *something* to be done. You as the patient are simply playing the 'sick' role; and part of that normal role involves seeking help and treatment for your sickness. You have been taught that this is your responsibility when you are in a sick, non-well or non-normal state. However, in the case of chronic pain, some of the usual rules have to change or the results can actually become dangerous. Doctors are, after all, only human; and when cast into the role of helper, they are responsive to the pressures of role-demands just like anybody else. Many doctors eventually give in to such pressure and prescribe more medication than they may feel should be prescribed, or they refer a patient for surgery in order to appease the pain-sufferer and end the frenzied demands for help. The tragedy is that the benefit of such measures is often negligible or only temporary, and when the latest 'solution' turns out to be another failure, the patient is back on the phone again or in the office demanding that something else or something more be done.

More tragic yet is the fact that often the cure is, indeed, worse than the disease. Excessive surgery for example, often leads to the creation of scar tissue which itself produces new pain. Excessive medication may lead to the Medication Trap and drug dependence. As the process continues, your doctor and his/her receptionist get more and more tired of you while you get more and more disillusioned and angry with the medical system. This hostility begins to be directed toward the medical profession in general. The chronic pain patient may finally leave this doctor and try another, but in time the same relationship will become established wherever the chronic pain patient goes for a 'cure'. Unfortunately this is a very common scenario for chronic pain patients and their doctors.

It does not, however, have to be the way things work. The main problem in this malfunctioning relationship is the *false* expectations that doctors *should* be able to *cure* or at least permanently relieve chronic pain. Often they simply can't. If you don't have one of the more clearly defined and well understood pain syndromes (which is usually diagnosed as such), you may have to accept this fact. If you have been through sufficient medical work-ups and especially if you have tried numerous 'solutions' which have failed, it may be time to accept that there are no medical solutions to cure *your* pain.

As stated earlier, what has been wrong with your doctor-patient relationship is that both you and your doctor have been following the rules and roles prescribed by the *usual* doctor-patient relationship, and these are not only ineffective but indeed can even be destructive in the case of chronic pain, where there may be no known physiological solution. (Remember that 'no physiological *solution*' does not mean 'no physiological *cause*'. Sometimes even when the cause is known, a cure is unknown.) You have probably been expecting your doctor to produce a rabbit from his magic bag of tricks. He may have tried to produce one, or several, but nothing has materialized. You have been assuming that it is possible to be completely cured of your pain and that, moreover, doing so is not *your* responsibility but your *doctor's*. As should be obvious by now, these ideas may be quite wrong.

If you have read and absorbed the message of this book so far, most likely you are beginning to see that although you may not be able to completely rid yourself of your pain, there are ways to *cope* with your pain and thereby make it more manageable. These coping strategies, however, must be largely *your* responsibility, not your doctor's.

Once you have accepted this premise, you and your doctor can try assuming new roles in the doctor-patient relationship. You will be shedding the usual 'sick role' with its demands to be helped or cured, and you will be ready to assume a 'rehabilitation role'. Rehabilitation means trying to live as independently and as normally as possible. Your doctor, in turn, can then take on the role of facilitator of your rehabilitation. As facilitator of your rehabilitation, your doctor will be able to take the part of your counsellor or consultant. You may consult him on such things as how quickly to increase exercises in your exercise programme, or he may help you set up the 'pain cocktail' described in Chapter 7. He should also become someone who encourages you in your progress. But the *responsibility* for implementing these coping, rehabilitation techniques must be *yours*.

If these are the new roles adopted by each of you, your focus will no longer be your pain or other problems, as in the past. In fact, there should be little need to talk of these things. The new focus will be, instead, upon your *adaptation*—your increasing activity, your new interests, your decreasing medication, your progress toward a new, more healthy and happy life. This new set of roles may, at first, be hard to adjust to, not only for you, but for your doctor as well. The doctor's office is, after all, where the patient usually tells his complaints and the doctor listens sympathetically. What is being suggested here is that visits to the doctor's surgery instead be oriented around the patient keeping the doctor up to date on his successes in overcoming chronic pain and its various, related 'traps', while the doctor offers encouragement and guidance. Doctors (and patients) often assume that if a patient isn't complaining any more, he no longer needs to come in for appointments. Of course, that is not always true. Indeed, as one starts along the difficult road to rehabilitation, regular contact with the doctor is as important as ever.

It is possible that you will find that this role-change is impossible for your doctor. Doctors are, after all, trained and usually practise the role of problem-*solver* as discussed above. If you do find your doctor unable to change, don't despair. There are other professionals, such as psychologists, who should also be able to help you, especially if they are specifically oriented toward the role of rehabilitation-facilitator. Psychologists can be found by consulting your local Pain Clinic (see Appendix). Many chronic pain patients are, unfortunately, reluctant to consult psychologists since they think that going to a psychologist implies that 'the pain is in your head' or imagined. This is an old-fashioned notion. Psychologists, these days, have become recognized as very helpful in applying their behavioural techniques to a range of medical problems. This book is, in fact, based on techniques derived from the relatively new areas of psychology called 'medical psychology' and 'behavioural medicine'. Because some of the principles of these new developments in psychology are not yet universally known, it is probably useful for you to familiarize your rehabilitation-facilitator, whoever he/she is, with this book, just to be sure.

Summary

1. The traditional doctor-patient relationship (doctor in the role of provider of cures and patient in the role of demander of solutions) is unlikely to work in the case of chronic pain problems. The doctor-patient relationship usually breaks down when the solutions do not work.

2. Demanding help from your doctor by frequent phone calls or visits, particularly demands for more medication and/or surgery, can be dangerous. If your doctor thinks you need more medication or surgery, he will recommend it on his own. Pressure from you may push him into a recommendation he is not sure about. Remember the old axiom: 'the cure can be worse than the disease' is very often true with chronic pain patients.

3. It is recommended that rather than assuming the 'sick role' for the patient and the 'curer of problems' role for the doctor, patients should take on a 'rehabilitation role' and the doctors, in turn, should become 'rehabilitation facilitators'. These roles involve a reversal of previous practices of the patient listing complaints and the doctor listening and then prescribing treatment. The doctor is encouraged instead to take on the role of listening and encouraging 'well', successful behaviour, such as how the patient is doing in his activity programme, how his reduction of medication is going or what plans the patient is making for the future. Doctors are urged to ask questions such as: 'Tell me what you've been doing lately', rather than 'tell me how you feel', so that the emphasis is directed away from, instead of toward, pain and problems. Only in this way can the doctor help the patient make the escape from the Chronic Pain Trap.

4. Psychologists may also serve in the role of rehabilitation-facilitators. They can usually be contacted through your local Pain Clinic (see Appendix). It is suggested that you familiarize your rehabilitation-facilitator with the principles of behavioural medicine found in this book.

5. The most important point of this chapter, however, is that solutions to your pain problem may not be available from your doctor or anyone else. The responsibility for controlling and managing your chronic pain problem is *yours*. It is only *you* who can get on top of your pain. No one else—not even your doctor—can do it for you.

5. How to Resume More Normal Activity

Ann, the woman introduced in Chapter 2 who had been caught in the Take It Easy Trap, began a programme to gradually build her activity level. After her doctor gave her the okay, she started walking, stair climbing, lifting, stationary bicycle exercises and car riding.

After establishing where to begin each activity by using baseline measurement, she chose daily goals with small daily increases (as explained in this chapter). She contracted to reward herself if she succeeded at her daily goals and to punish herself if she did not. While many people have days when they fail, Ann's daily goals and rewards must have been adjusted just right for her as she never missed a day. One of her favourite self-rewards was sleeping in late. A favourite bonus reward was a new article of clothing. Her family praised her progress and her husband showed his appreciation by bringing home special things she liked to eat, surprising her with flowers (for the first time in twenty years) and by sitting down with her for intimate talks rather than watching television (his usual activity in the evening).

Ann progressed from walking thirty-five steps to three kilometres a day. By the time she stopped exercising and returned to normal activity, she had progressed to three flights of stairs (up and down), two hours of car riding, lifting seven kilograms and riding eight kilometres on the stationary bicycle. By using task steps (as described in this chapter) she also worked herself back to doing normal housework. A few months later, she learned how to drive a car in order to have increased mobility. She took a part-time job as a cashier so that she could make her own spending money and, at the same time, resumed her bookkeeping classes. She persuaded her husband to take up square dancing and was proud that she could outdance him. Her family reported that her former grumpiness had been replaced by an improved mood and the return of her sense of humour. Ann had escaped the Take It Easy Trap.

If you carefully read the section on the Take It Easy Trap, discussed in Chapter 2, you will understand how inactivity has probably contributed to your problem. 'But,' you may say, 'I'm as active as I can be with my pain. Again and again I've tried to be active, but I *always* end up paying for it.' And it's probably true. The reason you end up paying for it is because you try to do *too much all at once*. Your muscles are weak from inactivity and when you do something strenuous it is not surprising that it causes you pain. The key words for this chapter are *gradual, systematic* and *regular*.

It is very important that you build activity *gradually* and *systematically*. You will need to begin a programme of exercise that will take time and you should plan to go about it regularly for at least the next several weeks. The exercises, however, needn't last forever. Once your activity level is more normal you will be able to apply your progress to more everyday practical activities. Many people do, in fact, continue their exercise programme indefinitely anyway, just because they learn to enjoy it. If approached correctly, exercise can be very satisfying and an excellent mood elevator.

A little later on in this chapter, several forms of exercise are suggested. You should determine which exercises are right for you and then check with your doctor to make certain that it is all right for you to work gradually on your chosen form(s) of exercise. It is possible that there will be some exercises that are inadvisable for medical reasons, but even if that is the case, you can be sure that there will be others that you *will* be able to work on. If you have difficulty finding exercises to suit you,

47

your doctor may be able to refer you to a physiotherapist whose training is in exactly this sort of thing.

The exercises outlined in this chapter are simple but practical ones such as walking, climbing stairs, riding in or driving a car, household tasks, or just sitting. They are things that many patients with chronic pain have gradually given up and now find difficult to do. You and your doctor or physiotherapist may decide on other types of exercise. The main thing that this chapter hopes to show you is the correct *method* for becoming more active. This method requires beginning with an easy starting place and taking small, gradual but consistent steps forward.

During the next several weeks you should consider yourself engaged in a training programme—a training programme to return you to normal. In the same fashion as an athlete, you will be retraining your body, your muscles and your mind. To assure success in this endeavour, it is strongly suggested that you negotiate 'contracts' with yourself. A sample of the type of contract you can make with yourself is shown on pages 58-9. Contracts are a good idea for several reasons:

1. They can detail specific daily goals.
2. They can provide consequences (rewards or punishment) for success or failure.
3. They can be excellent reminders or cues, especially if they are placed in a prominent place such as on the refrigerator door, on the television, or near the kitchen sink or bathroom wash basin.

For each exercise which you decide to incorporate into your programme you should determine your starting point. The best way to do this is by taking a 'baseline assessment' of your body's ability. Essentially, this means determining how much of any given exercise you can comfortably do at the present time. For the first three days of your exercise programme, you should plan specific times to try out an exercise, measuring how much you can do without pushing yourself. (Methods for measuring your effort will be explained in later sections describing specific exercises (see page 57).) Remember to do only as much as you can *without* causing your body any pain (either at the time of the exercise or later). Be conservative; don't overdo it. The point of the programme is to build your strength slowly and consistently. Overdoing it will cause you to have to stop your progress while you recover and you will ultimately be set back. Set-backs should be strenuously avoided. They only discourage you from trying further. This programme is structured to guarantee success by making the units of progress small enough so that they will be easy.

Eventually, you will be asked to choose rewards to give yourself when you succeed in meeting daily goals, and punishments to self-administer when you fail. The use of such programmed consequences has been found to be helpful in increasing overall success rates in exercise programmes. This will be discussed in greater detail below.

Once you have completed your three days of baseline assessment measures, it will be time to choose a beginning point for your programme, daily goals, daily rewards or punishments, as well as a regular schedule, referring to your **Activity Diary** (see page 32) for the best times. Each of the following sections suggests a beginning point based on your measurements. You will notice it is suggested that you begin slightly *below* your baseline levels. Again, this is to assure ease and success. Don't be tempted to start beyond this modest level. There is nothing to gain and much to lose by too ambitious a start.

Day-by-day goals are also suggested for each week. And each subsequent week's goals depend on how you performed in the previous week. Following this system helps to adjust your programme to your actual rate of progress. If you are usually succeeding, your programme is probably about right. If, however, you find you are consistently failing to meet your goals, your programme may just be too hard. However, there can be other reasons for failure. Some of the most common are related to the rewards and punishments you select for yourself. A later section of this chapter will discuss this problem in detail.

Suggestions for Activity Goal Setting

Each week's activity level should be based on your success rate in the previous week. Each person will begin and progress at a different rate. The important thing is not how fast you progress but that you make consistent, steady progress. Count the number of days you succeeded in the last week and then refer below.

Exercises:	Walking	Sitting	Stair climbing	Riding in a car
Week 1	1 step/day	1 min./day	1 stair-step/day	1 min./time
Subsequent Weeks				
If last week's success rate was 7 out of 7	2 steps/day	2 min./day	2 stair-steps/day	2 min./time
If last week's success rate was 6, 4 or 3 out of 7	1 step/day	1 min./day	1 stair-step/day	1 min./time
If last week's success rate was 2 or 1 days out of 7	1 step every 2nd day	1 min. every 2nd day	1 stair-step every 2nd day	1 min. every 2nd time

Your Exercise Programme Contract

There are several ways in which you can organize your exercise programme contracts. You may decide to do one exercise at a time with a separate contract for each, or you may decide to do two or more exercises concurrently with either separate contracts or one contract for all. People who have trouble thinking up daily rewards and punishments often find it easier to keep one contract for all exercises. The only drawback to such an approach is that you are requiring yourself to do *more* work to get the same reward (or avoid the same punishment). Therefore, if you adopt that system, you will want to be certain that the rewards and punishments are especially motivating ones! Finally, another pattern involves beginning with one exercise and in a couple of weeks or so adding a second and so on, revising old contracts, or adding new ones, as you prefer. How you make contracts with yourself and build your exercise programme is up to you. The important thing is to *do* it.

A good way to manage your self-contracting is to choose a regular time during the week to sit down and work out the next week's contract or set of contracts and stick to it. In effect, this means setting up a scheduled therapy hour with yourself. Consult your **Activity Diary** (page 32) to help you select a good time for this planning session. Many patients find it handy to do it on the weekend, perhaps after the children are in bed. Sunday evening often seems to be a particularly good time. Review your previous week's records, determine your success rate; then work out each day's goal for the next week, establishing daily rewards and punishments from a list you will draw up according to instructions given on pages 52-5.

Graphing Your Progress

Keeping track of your progress will be essential to your success. The best way to keep records is to chart them on a graph. Sample graphs of a walking exercise are shown on pages 62-3. You can easily prepare your own graphs basing them on these samples.

Keep a separate graph for each exercise. You will see that, across the bottom of the sample graph, the days are listed and grouped into weeks. Vertically along the left-hand column are the units of exercise measurement. (For example, the walking exercise is measured in number of steps.) You will need to work out the size of your exercise units so that, as you make progress, it will show up properly on your graph. You may wish to cheat slightly and start at the bottom of the graph with some figure above zero. This can help group units a bit better and allow progress to stand out more obviously. The sample graph on page 63 illustrates this technique.

Each day after you do your exercise, plot the correct point on your graph and connect the line from the last point. If you wish, make your graph in coloured pens, pencils or crayons so that the line of progress will stand out. As mentioned earlier, it is a good idea to hang your contract somewhere conspicuous in the house. This goes for your graph as well. Besides signalling to your family that you are working on overcoming your pain problem, they can serve as reminders or cues.

How to Select Rewards and Punishments

In your exercise programme you will be using rewards and punishments to help sustain your motivation. At first, patients often say, 'I don't need rewards and punishments; I'm not a child. I'll just use willpower,' or, 'They're silly. They won't really motivate me.' On the contrary, systems of reward and punishment are neither childish nor unrealistic. In fact, almost *everything* we do is related to the rewards or punishment we expect as a consequence. It's just another of those things that we don't often admit to ourselves. People work in order to receive their pay (a reward), simply because they enjoy their jobs (an intrinsic reward), or so that they won't be considered lazy by their families (an avoidance of punishment) and so on. People drive under the speed limit to avoid accidents (punishment) or traffic tickets (another form of punishment), or to receive praise from their families for being a good driver (reward). People are gentle, kind and considerate with their spouses at least in part so that they will receive reciprocal treatment (reward) and avoid resentment, anger and grouchiness in return (punishment). No matter what we may say, all of us enjoy being rewarded and desire to escape or avoid punishment.

Since this is a self-help programme you will be administering your own rewards and punishments in order to 'control' your own behaviour. Exercise programmes are never easy to do, as will be evident if you stop and think of the number of times you or others you know have begun on them in the past, only to quit soon afterwards. Why not resolve to do this one correctly by creating rewards and punishments which are powerful enough to help motivate you?

Rewards and punishments which do not really motivate you are not effective rewards and punishments for you. The only way to know whether they are right for you is to see whether they make you perform your exercises. If they do not, one of two things is wrong; either they are not strong enough, or they are not frequent enough. (Of course you have to apply them diligently for them to work at all.) A reward should be applied if you succeed at your task; a punishment if you fail. Before long you will find yourself succeeding all the time, provided you have planned your goals correctly and chosen effective rewards and punishments.

At this point, you may be saying to yourself, 'How can I find *daily* rewards and punishments for myself?' At first this task seems rather daunting, especially when every day has to be planned for. But it is really not so difficult. Perhaps the best way to see how it's done is to study pages 54-5 which gives examples of rewards and punishments that other people have found effective.

Sit down with your partner or family members and generate a long list of rewards and punishments. It is helpful to do this with someone else as they may be useful in getting you started, but it can, of course, also be done alone. You can start by referring to the examples and then being creative. Remember, though, that whatever you choose must be within your power to administer to *yourself*. While most people initially find this step rather hard, once they get started it becomes easier to think of things. Especially if two of you are working on it you should be able to generate at least twenty items in each list— one for rewards, one for punishments. And you can and should add to these over the weeks to come. Once you get into the swing of it, and you are succeeding regularly, the job of picking rewards and punishments can start being an enjoyable activity in itself.

Self-rewards and Punishments

Here are some suggestions for self-rewards and punishments which other chronic pain patients have used. Tick those which you think would be rewarding or punishing for *you*. You can use these ideas in your own list or make up an entirely new list.

Potential rewards

sleeping in late

staying up late

special food or drink (e.g. camembert cheese, chocolate, or champagne)—specify: _____

_____

extra helping of favourite—specify: _____

_____

back rub

hot bath

buying a special magazine—specify: _____

_____

breakfast in bed

playing cards

listening to the radio or to records or tapes

Potential punishments

getting up early

going to bed early

no television

not allowing certain food or drink—specify: _____

_____

not allowing self to watch news

getting breakfast

going out without make-up, socks, etc.

giving money to a political group you despise

cold shower

cleaning the kitchen

putting out the rubbish

not allowing self to read newspaper

being read to

time alone with someone

money toward some desired object (e.g. book, record, flowers or sport object)— specify: _____

_____

Your list:

_____

_____

_____

_____

Your list:

_____

_____

_____

_____

_____

_____

_____

_____

Increasing Walking

The first suggested task involves the increase of your ability to walk long distances. Walking is an excellent exercise for the body and necessary for so many activities. However, many chronic pain patients find they cannot walk very far at all. This is particularly, though not exclusively, true of people who suffer low back pain.

Walking is an important practical ability since it provides access to so many other activities which are avoided or given up if normal amounts of walking are difficult. Before deciding whether this section applies to you, ask yourself what you can no longer do or are restricted in doing as a result of pain caused by walking. If any of the following activities are involved, you may wish to participate in the walking programme: shopping, hiking, golfing, travelling, walking on the beach, or being employed in a job.

Baseline Assessment: Baseline assessment in this case refers to finding out how far you can currently walk with ease. During the first three days, walk only as far as you can *without*

55

causing yourself any pain (either during the walking or later). Plan to do this at a particular time of day—preferably the same time each day. Consult your **Activity Diary** to select a good time. You should count the number of steps you consecutively walk during the exercise itself (disregarding other walking which you would do anyway during the day). If you are fairly limited in your ability to walk, you can use your living room as your initial walking site. If walking is not too much of a problem, you may begin outside, weather-permitting; otherwise, use any indoor space, pacing back and forth, or join the local sports centre. No matter where you walk, be sure to count the number of steps. Steps are defined as each time a new foot is placed in front of you (right foot, one step; left foot, two steps, etc.). Record this on a graph as shown in the examples on pages 62 and 63 and as discussed under the section called 'Graphing Your Progress' (see page 51).

The Walking Programme:

Now you are ready to begin your programme. The first thing to do is to set yourself daily goals for each week. These goals should *gradually* increase the number of steps you walk and should be underwritten by the written contract that you make with yourself. Pages 58-9 show an example of such a contract. You will notice that the contract calls for a specific reward or punishment to follow your success or failure at accomplishing each goal. Don't omit the making of a contract. Contracts are not frivolous or unimportant to your programme. On the contrary, they are especially useful not only because they remind you exactly what you agreed to do and provide good cues (if placed in conspicuous places), but also they provide essential motivation through pre-arranged consequences for performing or not performing the tasks of your programme.

Follow the steps below to set up your walking programme:

Step 1: Select a starting goal by looking at your three days of baseline data and determining the *lowest* of these. Now subtract ten steps from the number and you have your first day's walking goal. If, for example, your lowest baseline day was 17 steps, begin at seven; if it was 53, begin with 43; if 419, begin with 409.

Step 2: Next, choose the number of steps that you wish to add on to your goal every day in the first week and enter it at the top of page 60 on the 'Walking Contract'. Also mark the sheet as 'Week 1'. For the first week, your goals should be fairly small. A one-step daily increase is recommended for Week 1.

Step 3: Next, decide when you will start your programme and write each day of the week and the date down along the left-hand column of the contract. Calculate your beginning daily walking goal as shown in Step 1 (your lowest baseline day minus ten steps) and write it under the first step of the daily walking goals in column two. For each subsequent day of the week, add your daily increase goal. Fill in the whole week. Next to each day under columns three and four, write in a daily reward and punishment from the list you have compiled. Some days may have the same reward or punishment as others, but it is important not to reward yourself with the same reward so often that you become satiated or tired of it since it then loses its rewarding value. The same is true of punishment. If the same one is given too often, you may get used to it, in which case it loses its punishing value.

Step 4: Sign the contract and date it. Remember that this means that you are committing yourself to follow all the terms of the contract, including the self-administering of rewards and punishments.

Step 5: Place the contract in a prominent place so that you will be reminded to follow it and to record whether you succeeded and whether you gave yourself the planned reward or punishment. The last two columns of the contract are for daily monitoring of yourself.

Step 6: Decide ahead of time *when* during the day you can do your walking. Referring back to your **Activity Diary** choose a time when other demands are low and before you are too tired. You don't want these things to become excuses. It is best to do

Example Walking Contract

I agree to try to meet my daily walking goal and not to give myself excuses for not doing so. If I meet my daily goal, I will reward myself with the daily reward. If I do not meet the goal, I will punish myself with the daily punishment.

My daily increase will be ___1___ steps/day for Week ___1___.

Day of week & date	Daily walking goal (in steps)	Daily reward	Daily punish-ment	√ if you succeeded & rewarded or punished self (R or P)	
Monday May 20	29	extra cup of coffee	can't read newspaper	√	R
Tuesday May 21	30	hot bubble bath	cold shower	√	R
Wednesday May 22	31	hamburger for lunch	no lunch	√	R
Thursday May 23	32	new magazine	no television until 5.00pm	√	R
Friday May 24	33	1 hour to read new magazine	go to bed at 9.00pm	√	R
Saturday May 25	34	hot bubble bath	cold shower	√	R
Sunday May 26	35	£5 for new parcel	get up at 7.00am	√	R

Bonus Reward: If I meet the goal for all seven days I will reward myself with *breakfast in bed*

I agree to do my walking at _*10.30 a.m*_ (time) each day and/or

after breakfast before 11.00 a.m

(other scheduling arrangement).

_____ *Joan Smith* _____ *18 May 1985*
(Signature)   (Date)

your walking at the same time each day and to make it into a routine. Choose either a specific time, such as 10.30 a.m., or choose a regularly occurring event for it to precede or follow, such as 'after breakfast'. It may be possible to use both systems in your plan, for example: 'I will do my walking each day after breakfast but no later than 10.30.' Whatever you decide regarding scheduling, write it at the bottom of your contract in the space provided.

Step 7: Immediately after completing each day's walk, mark your results on your contract. In conjunction with the contract, use your graph on page 64 to plot your progress. Record the days across the bottom of the graph and the number of steps up along the left-hand column. Each day, mark in the point for the number of steps completed for that day and connect the line from the previous day.

Step 8: You should now administer or plan to administer your reward or punishment. If it is possible to reward yourself immediately, do so. *Rewards given immediately work best.* If it is not possible to self-reward until later in the day, be sure to remind yourself that 'this reward is for accomplishing today's walking goal'. And regardless of when you give yourself a reward, you should mentally praise yourself. It is important for you to acknowledge your accomplishments. Think something to yourself such as: 'I'm proud of meeting my walking goal' or 'I'm doing well in my activity programme.' Self-praise is as important as more tangible rewards. Chronic pain sufferers often have the habit of giving themselves lots of self-criticism

Walking Contract

I agree to try to meet my daily walking goal and not to give myself excuses for not doing so. If I meet my daily goal, I will reward myself with the daily reward. If I do not meet the goal, I will punish myself with the daily punishment.

My daily increase will be_____steps/day for Week_____.

Day of week & date	Daily walking goal (in steps)	Daily reward	Daily punish-ment	√ if you succeeded & rewarded or punished self (R or P)	

Bonus Reward: If I meet the goal for all seven days I will reward myself with_____

I agree to do my walking at _____ (time) each day and/or

_____

(other scheduling arrangement).

_____   _____
(Signature)   (Date)

_____

but little self-praise. This is a good way to start reversing your negative thoughts about yourself.

If you fail to meet your daily goal, administer the punishment you have chosen for that day. Try to do it as soon as possible.

Whatever you do, don't give yourself excuses to get you out of your contract, even temporarily. Doing a good deal of walking for some other reason at another time during the day, for example, is *not* an acceptable excuse. The whole idea of this programme is that it is *regularly* and *systematically* getting you back in shape. Also *no* excuses are acceptable for 'forgetting' to give yourself rewards and punishments. Would the bank 'forgive' you if you 'forgot' to send in a loan repayment? Would the policeman overlook it if you 'forgot' about the speed limit? Well, this contract is just as important and just as firm.

Step 9: If you *do* succeed at meeting all of Week 1's walking goals, be sure to give yourself the extra prize specified as a Bonus Reward at the bottom of your contract. Make it a good one—you deserve it!

Step 10: You should tackle Week 2 in the same manner as Week 1. Make up a contract for the week, using Week 1 as your guideline. From now on, the success rate from each previous week should determine the goals you set for the next week. The table on page 50 suggests increases based on your success

Sample Walking Graph

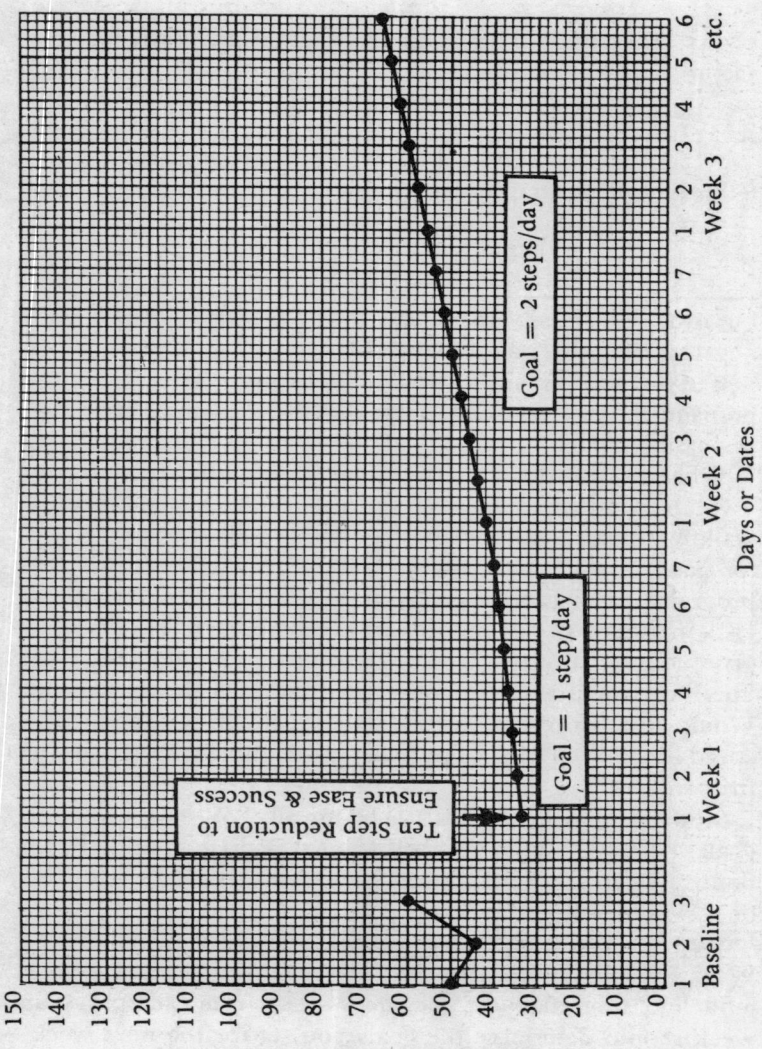

Sample Walking Graph
(with scale reduced to show up progress better)

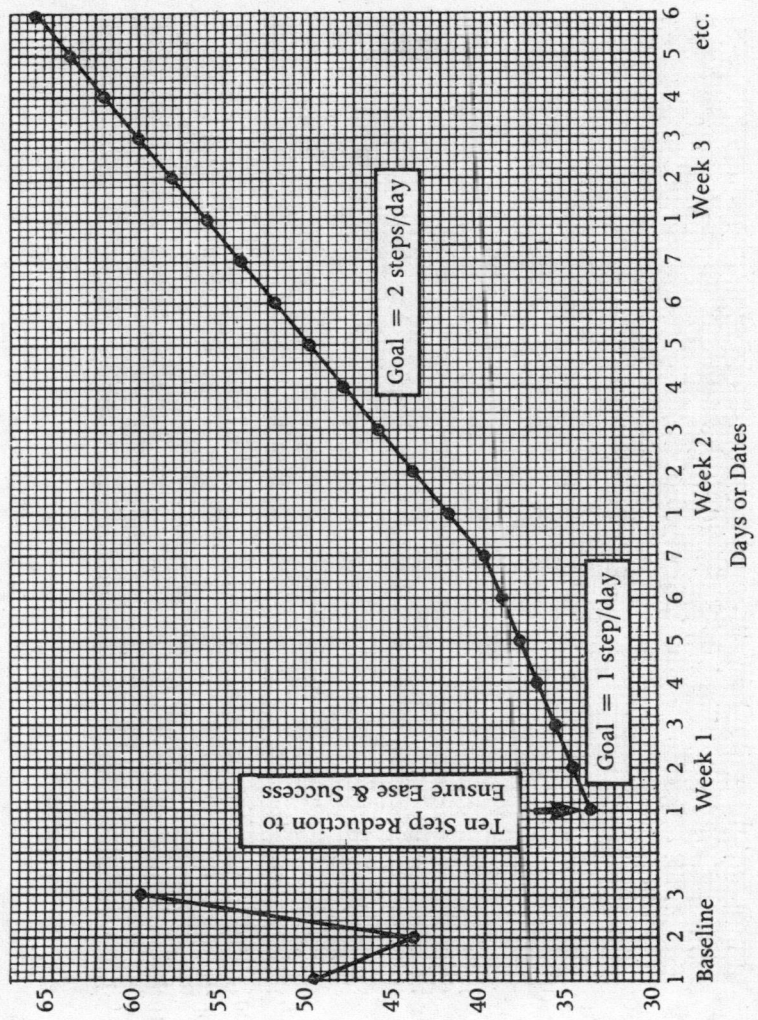

Walking Graph

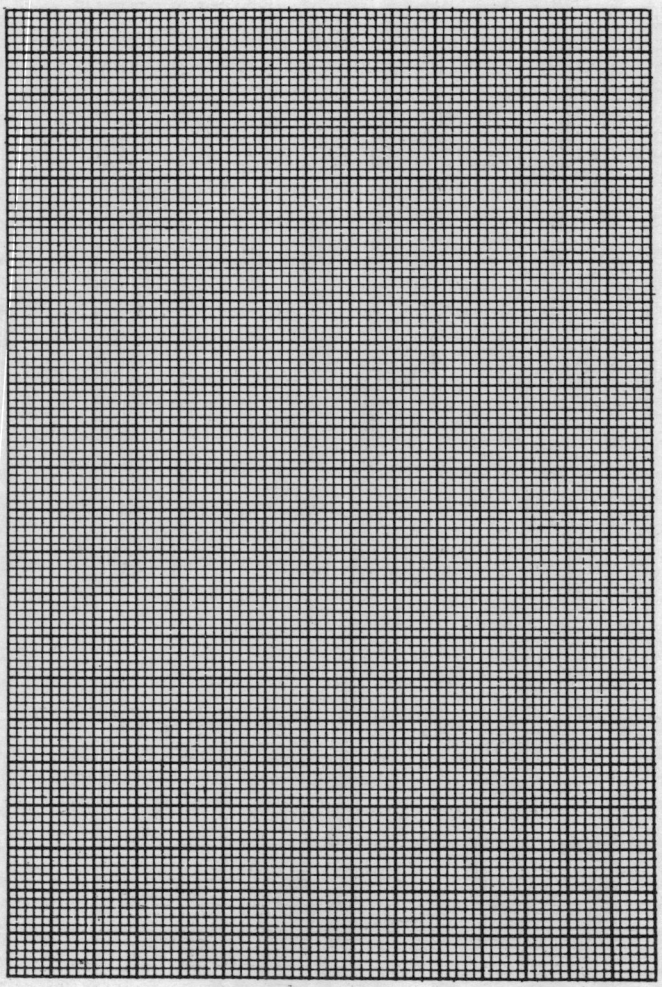

Days or Dates

Steps Walked/Day During Walking Exercise

rate. Count up the successes from the previous week and refer to this table to set the next week's goals. For example, if you succeeded in meeting all goals for Week 1, you may be ready to increase each day's goal by a slightly larger number of steps per day, for example, two steps increase per day in Week 2. However, if your success rate was less than perfect but you met your goal on at least three of the seven days, then plan to increase your daily goal by just one step per day in the next week. If you succeeded on less than three days, reduce your daily goal. You are probably getting ahead of yourself. You may want to make a one-step increase every second or third day. If you succeeded less than three days, it might also be a good idea to re-examine the strength of your self-rewards and self-punishments. They may need to be made stronger. Another possible problem is that you've neglected actually giving yourself rewards and punishments and you therefore have less motivation to succeed. This only illustrates that rewards and punishments really *are* necessary. Be sure to follow through next time.

Step 11: Each subsequent week, use the previous week's success rate as your guide in setting goals. Always refer to the table on page 50.

As chronic pain sufferers begin exercising regularly and their ability increases, they are often able to increase their goals by greater amounts. Thus, if you are succeeding consistently and wish to increase daily goals beyond two steps per day, do so, but don't go overboard. Work upward gradually. It is essential that you do not set goals so high that you fail consistently and end up discouraged. That only leads to quitting.

Another word of warning—*never exceed your daily goal!* Doing so risks set-backs. The most important aspect of the programme is its regularity. What will make you succeed is small daily advances—so small that they are not difficult to accomplish and success is relatively assured. These small gains inevitably add up to something worthwhile—your ability to be more active again!

Increasing Sitting Time

Sitting problems are most common among low-back pain sufferers, but may affect other chronic pain patients as well. This exercise will help you learn to sit for reasonable amounts of time. Sitting, after all, provides access to many other activities. You may wish to work on this exercise if you are unable to do any of the following: go out to dinner; go to a movie, concert, play or church; take a class; do a job which involves continuous sitting.

The same set of principles and steps applies in this exercise programme as were outlined for the walking programme. You will again be required to keep three days of baseline information, set daily sitting goals, sign a contract, reward and punish yourself and slowly increase daily goals until you are able to function normally again.

Baseline Assessment: The first three days will be a baseline phase to assess how long you can sit continuously (that is, without interruptions to stand or lie down) with ease and *without* causing yourself discomfort or pain during the sitting exercise or later.

Use the chair around the house which you find most *un*comfortable. (You will have to become accustomed to sitting in uncomfortable chairs: churches, football grounds and restaurants do not always have nice padded seats.) Find something enjoyable to do while sitting, preferably something active, such as letter writing, knitting, model building or playing cards. Avoid more passive activities, such as watching television or being read to. Then, while engaged in your chosen activity, time yourself for the next three days. Graph your sitting time on a graph as explained on pages 51-2 in the section entitled, 'Graphing Your Progress'.

The Sitting Programme:

Step 1: Set your first day's goal in the same way you did for walking. Choose the *shortest* time during your three days of baseline assessment; drop a few minutes from this and you have your beginning goal.

Step 2: Establish your goal for a daily increase. A reasonable daily increase for sitting time in the first week is one minute per day.

Step 3: Fill out the sitting contract for the first week. Write in each day's goal, reward and punishment and a bonus reward.

Step 4: Do your sitting exercise at regular, pre-arranged times in the day. Use your **Activity Diary** to help you set up your schedule. Remember to keep busy doing something while you sit. Being involved in some activity will make the time pass faster and keep you from thinking about your problems. If you don't have something readily available to do, make the effort to try something new. Suggestions for activities while sitting are: letter writing, knitting, crocheting, mending, model building, painting, creative writing, embroidery, playing a musical instrument, weaving, spinning, macrame, leather work, pottery, jewellery-making or toy-making, or reading a magazine or newspaper. If all else fails, go to a novelty or arts and craft shop and see what catches your eye.

Step 5: Record your progress daily on both your contract and your sitting graph.

Step 6: Administer to yourself your daily reward or punishment. Remember to give yourself mental praise if you succeed.

Step 7: Each subsequent week when you prepare your contract, use the previous week's success rate for your guide. Refer to the table on page 50 to plan your goals. However, be reminded that the important thing is to make *small* but *daily* advances—so small that you can easily succeed. Over time, they will amount to substantial accomplishments allowing you to engage in many of your old activities once again.

Sitting Graph

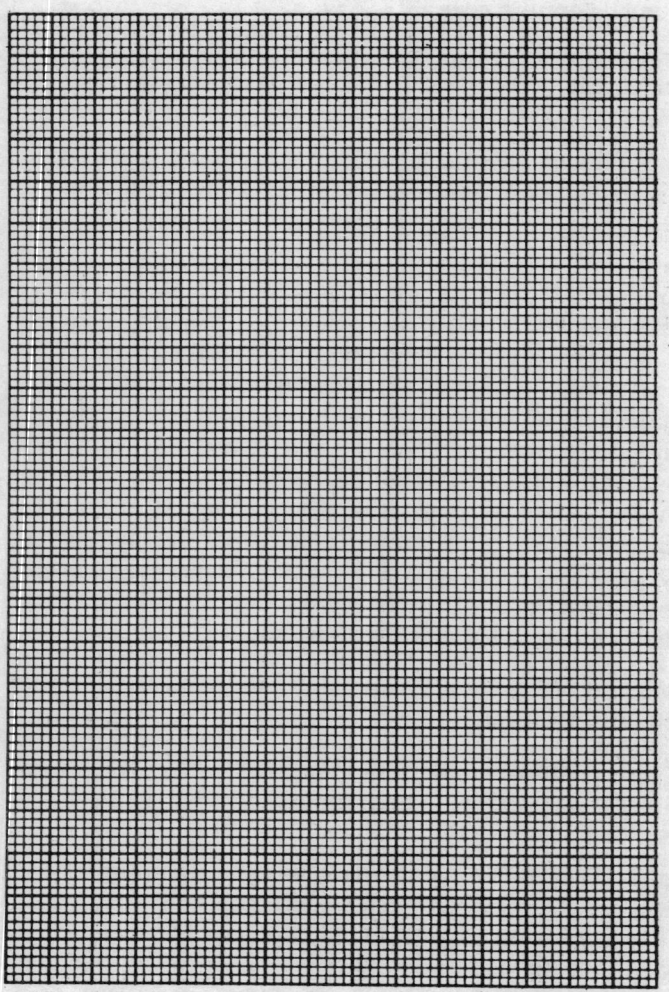

Days or Dates

Time Spent Sitting/Day

Sitting Contract

I agree to try to meet my daily sitting exercise goal and not to give myself excuses for not doing so. If I meet my daily goal, I will reward myself with the daily reward. If I do not meet the goal, I will punish myself with the daily punishment.

My daily increase will be _____ for Week _____.

Day of week & date	Daily goal (in length of time)	Daily reward	Daily punish-ment	√ if you succeeded & rewarded or punished self (R or P)	

Bonus Reward: If I meet the goal for all seven days, I will reward

myself with _____

I agree to do my sitting exercise at _____ (time)
each day and/or

_____

(other scheduling arrangement).

_____   _____
              (Signature)   (Date)

Stair Climbing

Many chronic pain patients are limited by an inability to climb
stairs. Once again, this is most common among patients with
low-back pain. If you feel this problem limits your mobility,
either at home or when going out, this may be an exercise for
you to work on. You must, of course, have a set of stairs
available at home or close by to undertake easily this programme, but even a few steps can do the trick.

Begin by taking baseline measurements for three days. How
many steps can you climb up and down without interruption
and *without* causing yourself pain (at the time or later)? On
three consecutive days, try this climbing test, counting the
steps and recording the results on one of the graphs provided.

Once you have completed these measurements, you will be
ready to negotiate a contract with yourself using one of the
contract forms. These are the steps that you should follow:

Step 1: Choose a starting point for the first day of your
exercise programme. A good starting point is about three steps
less than your lowest baseline day.

Step 2: Set a goal for your daily increase. Remember to keep
it small. One additional step per day is a good rate for Week 1.

Step 3: Choose daily rewards and punishments for yourself
from the lists that you've made up. Write these, along with a
bonus reward, into your contract.

Step 4: After signing and dating your contract, place it along
with your graph in a prominent place.

Stair Climbing Graph

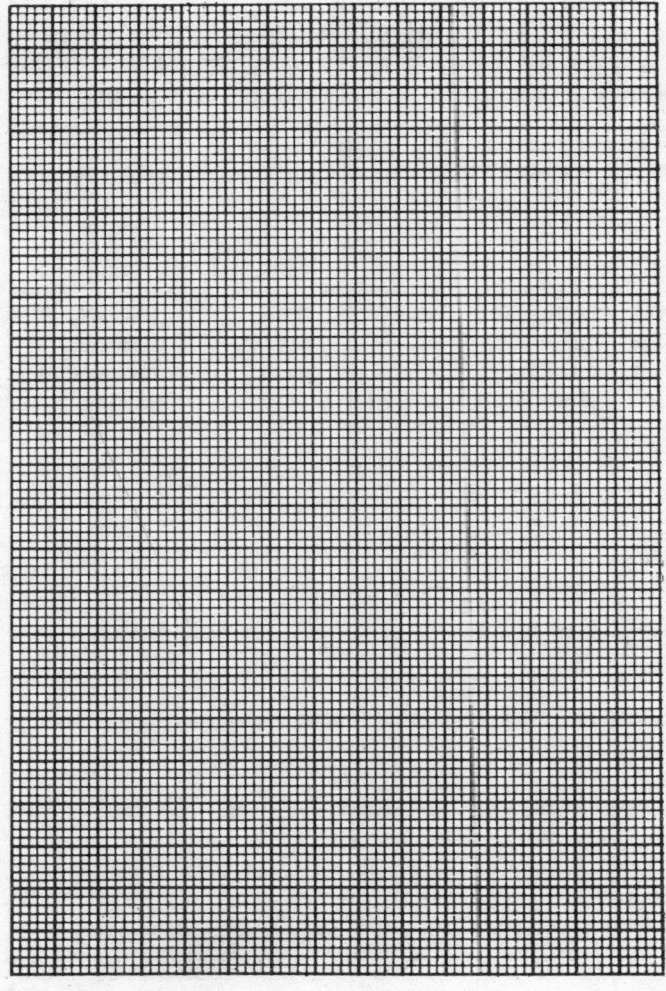

Days or Dates

Stairs Climbed/Day

Stair Climbing Contract

I agree to try to meet my daily stair climbing exercise goal and
not to give myself excuses for not doing so. If I meet my daily
goal, I will reward myself with the daily reward. If I do not
meet the goal, I will punish myself with the daily punishment.

My daily increase will be _____ steps/day for
Week_____.

Day of week & date	Daily goal (in number of stairs)	Daily reward	Daily punish-ment	√ if you succeeded & rewarded or punished self (R or P)

Bonus Reward: If I meet the goal for all seven days, I will reward myself with _____

I agree to do my stair climbing at _____ (time) each day and/or

_____

(other scheduling arrangement).

                   (Signature)   (Date)

Step 5: Begin your exercise programme, reserving a regular time for it each day when distractions are at a minimum. Use your **Activity Diary** to pick the best times.

Step 6: Immediately after completing your exercise each day, record your results on the contract and on the graph.

Step 7: As soon after the exercise as possible, administer to yourself your reward or punishment, whichever you have earned. If you have succeeded, don't forget to praise yourself as well. After all, you are accomplishing something of which you can be proud. Sticking to an exercise programme really is something terrific.

Step 8: Each week, re-negotiate your contract. Remember to set each week's goal according to the previous week's success rate. You can refer to the table on page 50 as a guideline.

Increasing Ability to Ride In or Drive a Car

Many chronic pain patients report they are unable to ride in a car for very long distances. Others report they are unable to drive. Either of these problems can severely restrict your ability to get around and do things normally. Inability to drive or ride long distances in a car can be tackled in the same way as walking, sitting or stair climbing problems. Learning to do it is

73

Controlling Chronic Pain

Car Riding Contract

I agree to try to meet my daily car riding exercise goal and not
to give myself excuses for not doing so. If I meet my daily goal,
I will reward myself with the daily reward. If I do not meet the
goal, I will punish myself with the daily punishment.

My daily increase will be _____ for
Week_____.

Day of week & date	Daily goal (length of time)	Daily reward	Daily punish-ment	√ if you succeeded & rewarded or punished self (R or P)	

Bonus Reward: If I meet the goal for all seven days, I will reward

myself with _____

I agree to do my car riding at_____ (time)

each day and/or

_____

(other scheduling arrangement).

_____   _____

(Signature)   (Date)

merely a matter of gradually increasing your body's tolerance for the activity.

Begin by taking baseline measures for three days. Since they involve having a car available, there may be more difficulty in scheduling these testing sessions. You may have to work out with your partner or family member which days the car is available, and if required, which days they are able to drive for you. Ideally, your baseline measurements should be taken on three consecutive days, but adjustments may have to be made according to the situation. Baseline, in this case, is measured by how many minutes you can drive or ride without getting out of the car and *without* causing pain at the time or later—only as much as you can do comfortably. Driving or riding during these baseline sessions (and during the exercise programme which follows) should be just for the sake of driving: that is, no errands, pick-ups, deliveries or anything of the sort. Moreover, your route should be planned to keep you close to home so that you can end a session whenever you choose. During baseline you may wish to just go around the block a few times. If you have not been in a car for a while, this may be a particularly good idea for getting you back into the swing of things. It is important to very gradually ease yourself back into the hassles of driving—traffic, highway speeds, poor weather conditions—as well as into the exercises themselves.

Car Riding Graph

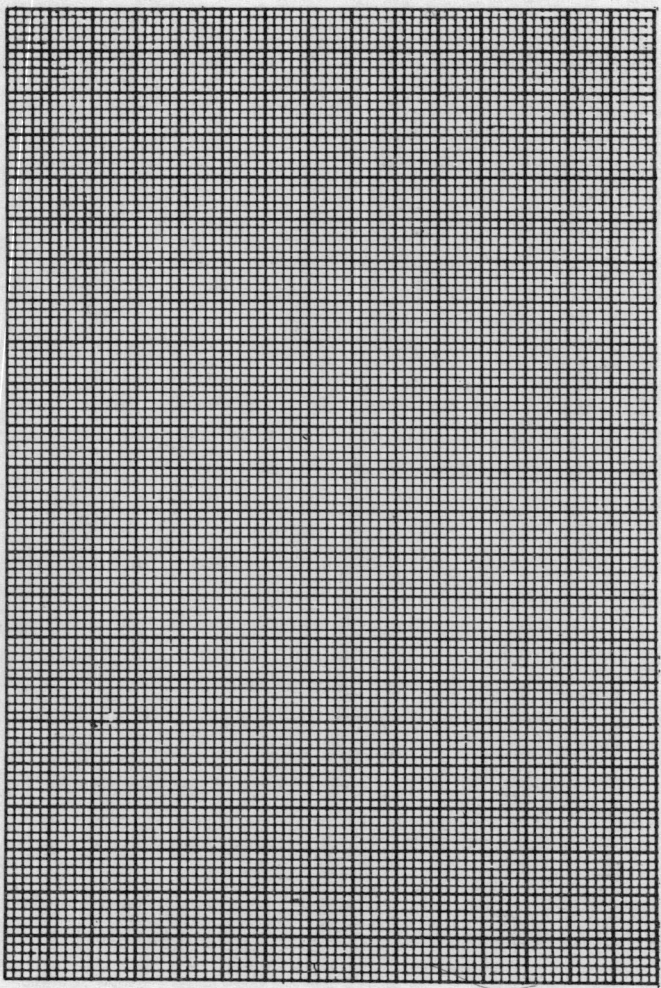

Days or Dates

Time Taken/Day

If you were once able to drive, you can probably work on this exercise programme entirely on your own. All you need is the car. If, however, you are unable to drive, you may need your partner's or another family member's help, since someone will have to drive while you practise riding. If both riding and driving are problems, you may wish to start with riding, and only after your body has built up a good tolerance for that activity, go on to the driving programme. At any rate, you will probably have to do some negotiation for the car and perhaps a driver. Since arrangements may not be possible every day, you will have to piece together the best schedule that you can. But you should do your best to work on this exercise at least three times a week. If you work on it fewer than that, your increases will mount up very slowly and you are likely to be discouraged. Of course, the more days you can arrange to practise, the better.

Once you have taken baseline measures, negotiate a contract with yourself. Set goals for each planned drive or ride; work out daily rewards and punishments as well as a bonus reward for the week. Plan to begin by driving a few minutes less than your lowest baseline day. A good goal for daily increase in the first week is one minute per day.

As you ride or drive, enjoy yourself. Have a look around, take new routes, play the radio, or chat with your partner. Do *not*, however, discuss how you feel or talk about your pain. Read ahead to Chapters 8 and 9 if you find yourself doing this.

Remember that driving during this exercise time is in addition to any other driving or riding which you may do during the day. Ignore what you may have done in addition. It shouldn't be used as an excuse to avoid or reduce your regularly scheduled driving or riding exercise.

Since you may have to rely on someone else to help you with this exercise, problems arise if the other person backs out. This exercise should be considered important and, ordinarily, it should take precedence over other activities which might come up. This is why it is negotiated ahead of time at the beginning of each week and then set down in writing. But, if something really unavoidable does come up, renegotiate an alternate time as soon as possible. Your learning to ride in or drive a car again for longer distances will pay off for the whole family!

If your partner is also reading this book, he will be more aware of why keeping to the terms of your contract is so important for *both* of you. But remember that it is also important for you to make his helping worthwhile. Let him know you appreciate the assistance. Be pleasant and enjoyable to be with; do something nice and special in return to show your thanks. After all, your exercise activity may have to take place after a long day or it may replace something else your partner enjoys doing. Show you appreciate it.

Increasing Other Exercises

There are any number of other exercises which you can work on in the same manner—first carefully assessing your starting point, then working out daily goals, weekly contracts and daily rewards and punishments. You may choose to work on as many as you feel comfortable with, either one after the other or together. But remember to consult your doctor or physiotherapist first, to help you determine which exercises might be most advantageous and to be sure that none could be harmful to your health. A visit to the physiotherapist can, in fact, be a particularly good starting place for devising new exercises especially suited to your needs. Often the physiotherapist can suggest and show you how to do various specific exercises such as let-backs, half knee-bends, leg-raising and arm-raising exercises or others which are beyond the scope of this book, but which can also be done at home in a self-help programme of this type. Just apply the formula—an easy beginning point, small increases, daily goals, self-contracting and self-administration of daily rewards and punishments. One word of caution though—in some of the more strenuous exercises, such as let-backs and half knee-bends, you may not be able to increase your goal on a daily basis. Instead you may wish to work out an increase every second, third, fourth or fifth day. This is fine. What is important is regular exercise, gradually increasing. The rate of increase should be small enough that you can succeed; otherwise it's up to you.

Other, more natural exercises, such as swimming, bicycle riding, jogging, golf, tennis or other ball games are also excellent. You may not be able to do all of them. Again, it's best to check out your plans with your physician. But you can nearly always find a sport that is safe and suits you. Swimming, for example, is one that almost everyone can do. Perhaps you will wish to set up swimming times for yourself at a local pool. You can count strokes.

A stationary exercise bicycle, while it may be somewhat expensive to purchase, provides an excellent alternative for exercise which can be programmed according to the pattern outlined in this book. You can determine your baseline, begin a few units below your baseline and give yourself weekly goals to increase the number of units achieved. Of course, check with your doctor before starting.

For more information on possible exercise programmes, see the section entitled 'Exercise' at the back of the book under 'Further Reading'.

Increasing Housework

Housework can be tackled in exactly the same way as other exercises. You may wish to choose one aspect of housework to work on first and gradually add others. Some common housework tasks are suggested in the list on page 80. You can probably think of others to add to your own list. Using the book's list as a starting point make a list of tasks which you 'Can do easily' and 'Can't do easily' using the worksheet labelled 'Housework List' on page 81. The things that you write down should be tasks relevant to *your* housework and *your role* (as you would like to see it) in the household.

Common Housework Tasks

Housework tasks vary from household to household. Tick the tasks which are performed with some regularity in your household. Add to your own list any which are not listed here. This can serve as a basis for your worksheet.

Preparing breakfast

Preparing lunch

Preparing dinner

Setting the table

Clearing the table

Washing dishes (by hand or loading and unloading dishwasher)

Dusting

Grocery shopping

Making beds

Vacuuming

Scrubbing floors

Cleaning the bathroom

Washing clothes

Ironing clothes

Folding clothes

Picking up toys, clothes, etc.

Others

_____

_____

_____

_____

_____

_____

_____

_____

_____

_____

_____

_____

_____

_____

_____

Housework List
and Task Steps Worksheet

Can do easily	Can't do easily

Target task:

_____

Task steps:

1. _____ 8. _____

2. _____ 9. _____

3. _____ 10. _____

4. _____ 11. _____

5. _____ 12. _____

6. _____ 13. _____

7. _____ 14. _____

15. _____   18. _____

16. _____   19. _____

17. _____   20. _____

Now choose a task from the 'Can't do easily' part of the list (preferably one of the easier tasks) and break it down into small task steps. As an example, let's take making beds.

Target task:
Making the three
beds in the house

—John's bed
—Mary's bed
—Our bed

Steps:
John's bed:
 1. Straightening the bottom sheet
 2. Fluffing the pillows
 3. Straightening the pillow cases
 4. Placing the pillows in the correct position
 5. Pulling the top sheet into place
 6. Tucking the top sheet under the mattress
 7. Pulling the blanket into place
 8. Tucking the blanket under the mattress
 9. Arranging the bedspread over the blanket
10. Tucking the bedspread under the pillows
Mary's bed:
Steps 11-20 (same steps as 1-10 above)
Our bed:
Steps 21-30 (same steps as 1-10 above)

This example describes the steps I go through when I make a bed. You may do it differently. But, however you do it, it is necessary for you to work out the process step by step. Notice how small the steps in the example are and avoid making yours any larger.

Now, using this method for approaching activities, take a baseline assessment of yourself. Do only as much as you know won't cause you pain; that is, stop before the activity becomes painful—now or later. If this leaves the bed half-made, leave it that way. Someone else can finish it.

Once you have carried out your baseline assessment, you will be ready to negotiate a contract with yourself. First, work out a beginning point. Drop back one or two steps from your lowest baseline level. If you were unable to do *any* of the task steps, choose Step 1 as your initial goal. Then establish daily goals for yourself. You might, for example, decide to progress forward one step every other day or every third day. Leave beds unfinished if you are midway to finishing them. The purpose of this programme is to *retrain you, not* to get the house sparkling. In time, you will be able to finish making beds. And in any case, they have probably gone unmade or have been made by someone else up until now, so continue that system until you reach the end of your step sequence.

Set yourself daily rewards and punishments and graph your progress. Start by putting the steps of the sequence beginning with Step 1 at the bottom of the left hand side of your graph. In the bed-making case, steps 1-30 would be listed in ascending order up the left hand margin of the graph. Days would be placed along the bottom. Graph the highest step attained each day.

Since task step sequences for housework are not as easy to quantify as our other exercises, and since it is sometimes hard to make the task steps of equal difficulty, you may find some steps in the sequence easier than others. If one step appears too hard, analyse it and break it down further into *smaller* steps. As someone once said: 'The only way to eat an elephant is one bite at a time.'

Now it's time to break other household tasks into task steps. Task steps are usually quite individual to your method of doing things, your house, your appliances and the size of your family. Using the **Task Steps Worksheet** on pages 81-2 choose a household task and try breaking it into smaller steps or units.

Imagine yourself doing the task and divide each separate set of movements into a separate step.

Many patients find it especially hard to leave household chores half-done. The source of trouble lies in your expectations for yourself or in your definition of a task or both. You may feel, for instance, that you will be failing at your vacuuming task if you don't vacuum the whole house. Of course, the problem is with your definition of success and your definition of what the vacuuming task is all about. You should do your best to redefine both success and the task itself in terms of your contract agreements. That means not thinking in terms of what you used to be able to do, or what you hope to be able to accomplish later on, but instead, focussing on the achievement of programmed steps in the context of an overall effort at self-help. You'll be doing better at your important job—getting back to normal—if you work gradually and systematically and don't overdo it. Overdoing it only leads to set-backs. Leave the other half of the room unvacuumed. You can always work on it again the next time vacuuming is scheduled on your contract.

Increasing Other Types of Work Tolerance

Of course, there are many forms of work other than housework. But the same techniques can be used to build tolerance for any of them, such as gardening, sewing, odd jobs, paying jobs or volunteer jobs. Work is an important part of everybody's life. Indeed, as discussed in the 'Take It Easy Trap' section of Chapter 2, a lack of meaningful work can be destructive to both your physical and mental health. At the same time, however (as will be discussed later on in Chapter 11 under 'An Unhappy Job Situation'), work which is intolerable or hated can also adversely affect your health. What this chapter will address, however, is work that you *want* to do, work you can be proud of and from which you can gain a sense of accomplishment. You may wish to skip ahead and read the section of Chapter 11 called 'An Unhappy Job Situation' before reading on if you now have or have had a job which you hated and which you feel may have affected your well-being.

Using the form below, make a list of the work goals that you would like to set for yourself. If you want to mow the lawn or wash the car, write it down; if you want to return to being a secretary, salesman, accountant or whatever else, write this down including the number of hours per week you hope to work (8, 24, 40, etc.). If you want to do volunteer work at a child care centre, a home for pensioners or with a fire fighting brigade, write these sorts of things down as well. The set of procedures to get your work tolerance programme going will be essentially the same as in the previous programmes. Find out, by testing yourself, how much of the chosen work activity you can currently do before you get into trouble with pain.

Work Goals

At Home	Volunteer Work	Competitive Employment

Measure it in terms of minutes, hours or specific units (such as number of rows of grass cut or percentage of car washed). You can then select for your training programme a beginning amount slightly below your baseline level.

Make a contract with yourself. Decide how often you want to engage in the work activity. Set slightly increasing goal requirements for yourself. Programme and give yourself rewards and punishments.

As discussed under the previous section on increasing housework, you may have to leave jobs partially unfinished. You can always do some more of it the next time or let someone else in the family finish it until you have worked your way up to being able to complete the whole task in one session. Unfortunately, however, we often worry about what the neighbours are going to think. To the outsider, it may seem a bit odd that the lawn is being left only partly mowed or the car only partly washed. But there are ways to deal with this sort of worry. First, if you do the task often enough, it should be obvious to anyone that you are not leaving jobs undone; you are doing them conscientiously and thoroughly, but progressively. Moreover, your neighbours may be more than happy to see that you are engaging in work activities again and that you are doing better and better at them. Another way to approach the problem is to forget about the neighbours, no matter what they think. After all, do the opinions of others really matter? Are they really worth worrying about and are they more important than your and your family's health and happiness? Why not just refuse to worry about what others may think?

It is sometimes possible to work your way gradually back to work at a paying job. Some companies are willing to negotiate a partial return schedule so that you can come to work again on a gradually increasing basis. If this is not possible, you may be able to increase your work tolerance yourself to an acceptable level by simulating your old job and working away at it gradually. For example, if you are a secretary, you can set up and do typing at home on a gradually increasing basis; if you are a maintenance worker, you can start on house and yard work; if you are a teacher, you can begin by doing some volunteer teaching. Sometimes patients can find part-time work which helps them rebuild their strength for general work tolerance. Volunteer work can do the same thing for you. In fact, many hospitals, schools, nurseries, homes for senior citizens and other institutions *need* volunteers. Often you can determine your own hours, increasing the time you spend as you progress. Volunteer work can serve other purposes as well. It can provide you with something else on which to focus your thoughts besides your own problems. It can be immensely satisfying and allow you to feel useful and worthwhile through contributing to someone else's happiness.

Summary

This chapter has been devoted to suggesting a method for increasing activity. The method involves determining what your body is currently *able* to do by baseline assessment (counting and recording how many units of a given exercise or activity that you can perform *without* pain). You work out your starting point by beginning a little lower than your baseline level and then determine your daily goals for yourself. Using the method of self-contracting, you establish ahead of time your daily goals for a week at a time and plan daily rewards and punishments to be self-administered for success or failure. Each day when you finish your exercises, you record your progress on a graph for each exercise. Finally, you give yourself your rewards and praise yourself for meeting your goals. Each week the contract is re-negotiated with new daily goals, based on your success rate the previous week. And you can apply this system to just about any exercise or activity you choose. A few practical exercises have been outlined here in detail—walking, sitting, stair climbing, driving or riding in a car, housework, recreational exercises and work tolerance. But patients are reminded in all cases to check out their plans with their doctor or physiotherapist. Additional reading on the subject of increasing activity levels is suggested; appropriate sources of information are listed on pages 189-202.

By using the method discussed here you *can* slowly work your way back to normal. It has worked for hundreds of other chronic pain patients and it can work for you!

6. Fighting Off the Depression of Chronic Pain

The feeling that you have little or no control over what happens to you is a common cause of depression. This is why depression often accompanies the condition of chronic pain. Patients may feel that their doctors, the pain itself or the pain medication have some control over their lives, but that they themselves are helpless to influence the things that determine their future. Chronic pain patients often fall victim to pessimism. They feel that pain is ruining their lives and that there is nothing they can do about it. Of course, this book suggests that you *can* get both your pain and depression under control, and that you *can* learn to cope.

The most common symptoms of depression are: loss of energy; lethargy; loss of interest in activities which you previously enjoyed; feelings of failure, guilt or self-blame; frequent crying; feelings of despair; loss of appetite; disturbed sleep patterns; or suicidal thoughts or wishes. Not everyone has all of these, but if some of these sound familiar, you may be depressed. And if you are, it is worth doing something about it. Depression has been shown to intensify pain, as well as vice versa, so that patients find themselves on a downward spiral of lower mood states and more intense pain.

Controlling Chronic Pain

Of course, you *can* control your pain, and you *can* control your life. The suggestions in this book are aimed at helping you to start toward this goal. Just by purchasing and reading this self-help book, you have already taken a first step toward regaining control of your environment, your body and your moods; and that's what fighting depression is all about. Being able to structure your environment to provide you with enough positive rewards and to minimize aversive experiences gives you the motivation to keep trying. Not receiving enough positive experiences or receiving too many negative ones kills that motivation. If you have been caught in the Chronic Pain Trap, chances are that you feel you have been having too many negative experiences and not enough positive ones.

This book is designed to give you suggestions for taking control of your environment and yourself. It attempts to show you how to minimize negative experiences (like pain and depression) and maximize positive ones (such as your assets, pleasurable experiences and emotions). If, however, you feel too depressed to begin work on your own, or if you feel suicidal, then you should seek professional help immediately. You can contact a psychologist or psychiatrist by calling your nearest Pain Clinic (see Appendix). Most towns also have Crisis Centres—The Samaritans or Nightline—which run 24-hour telephone services; these telephone numbers can be found in the telephone book or by asking Directory Enquiries.

Learning to Like Yourself Better

It is bad business not to like yourself, but many people don't. They focus on the negative aspects of themselves to the exclusion of any thought about their positive assets. One of the problems with this kind of thinking is that it often snowballs. The more negative things one focuses upon, the more pessimistic one feels. It then becomes all the more difficult to think about anything positive. People who are depressed often become very fixed upon a certain series of faults that they find in themselves. They may spend a good deal of their time thinking or talking about these negative aspects and they can therefore seldom, if ever, admit that they are really very nice people. It is as if they had on glasses which excluded the beautiful, good things in the world and themselves, and only showed them the bad aspects. Their attention and perception focuses on what is bad, wrong, or negative. This mode of thinking, which seems to come with depression, actually works to maintain the depression; it eventually spreads beyond the self and colours the way in which the whole world is seen. It's pretty difficult to feel good when all you can see is the gloomy side of the picture.

To create a shift in mood, a change has to be made in one's thinking. To become *un*depressed, negative attitudes and self-statements have to be changed. You have to emphasise and start focussing on what's good about you, on your successes, *and* you have to *stop* dwelling upon your failures and problems.

You can begin this change of direction by making a list of your positive attributes. What things are good about you? What do you like about yourself? Of what are you proud? Write down everything that comes to mind, no matter how small some of the things may be. A worksheet is provided on page 92.

All too often in our culture we are discouraged from praising ourselves or even from *noticing* our good points. This is really sad. Patients, for this reason, sometimes feel guilty, or at other times, ridiculous about working on lists of personal assets. But what kind of craziness is it that has been perpetrated upon us that we are afraid or reluctant to recognize ourselves as nice, likeable, attractive human beings? There is not only nothing wrong with doing this, there is something wrong with *not* doing it. We are limiting and restricting our pleasure and reinforcing our negative view of ourselves and our world. So, break free of those restrictions and start by making up this list.

Positive Attributes List

_____

_____

_____

_____

_____

_____

_____

_____

_____

_____

_____

_____

_____

_____

_____

_____

_____

_____

_____

_____

_____

Begin your list with notes about your physical appearance. Even if you don't consider yourself attractive, think about your best features. Everybody has them. What physical features do you like about yourself (eyes, hair, hands, fingernails, eyelashes, a well-placed mole, a hairy chest, small feet, good shoulders, even teeth)? Keep trying until you come up with several. Remember that they needn't be things universally endorsed by our society. People can like features about themselves which are not considered beautiful by the usual, confining standards (large, strong hands, thick eyebrows, a full rounded figure, spectacles, a distinctive birthmark or scar). These things may make us interesting or individual. *Stop* repeating to yourself anything that you consider a flaw. This exercise is meant to help you focus on the good things.

Next, give some thought to the personality traits which you are proud to have (friendliness, stability, a good sense of humour, dependability, generosity, sensitivity, ability to love, neatness, even temper, etc.). Just as in the case of physical features, there may be personality traits that you like in yourself which don't conform exactly with the cultural norms (unpredictability, stubbornness, being a penny-pincher, being remote or aloof, being emotional). If you like these aspects about yourself, write them down too. These examples are only provided to illustrate the type of thing being asked of you; it is up to you to come up with traits or attributes which fit you.

Which of your intellectual aspects do you think are good (common sense, ability with figures, good intuition, being well-read, open-mindedness, expertise in one or more topics, etc.)?

Finally, list all your skills (cooking, parenting, singing, playing an instrument, playing chess, telling jokes, arguing or debating, typing, woodworking, or some other job skill or craft, etc.).

Keep working on your list until you have at least fifteen things written down. Then try to add to it each week.

Now that you have generated a list of positive, attractive,

likeable things about yourself, the trick is to practise thinking about them. Notice your nice nose or attractive eyes when you look in the mirror. Take pride in your sense of humour when you make someone laugh. Give yourself a little pat on the back when your child confides in you or snuggles up on your lap. Enjoy something delicious you made to eat; notice how good it is and how it pleases others.

Another good idea is to practise making positive statements about yourself to yourself. One way to go about this is to use a stack of small file cards as reminders. Jot down one item from your list of assets on each card. Then keep the cards handy in a pocket, drawer or handbag. Several times each day, pull them out and read through them. Some people do this along with some frequently occurring event, for example every time you have a cup of coffee or light up a cigarette. Pairing it with some other activity assures that you will do this review regularly. The cards are small and can be stacked and carried anywhere, and they're easy to add to as you think of new things.

There is one more activity you should add to your programme of self-appreciation. Near the end of each day, review the day's accomplishments and give yourself the credit you deserve. Say to yourself: 'I'm proud of myself today because: I didn't mention pain to anyone today; I succeeded in my exercise programme; I remembered to praise Johnny for making his bed; I finished reading my library book; I made Ann happy by remembering our anniversary,' or whatever. Try to think of at least one statement each day; there will always be something, and often many things, to praise yourself for after any given day, especially if you are putting the other aspects of this self-help programme into effect.

What is being suggested is that you work on self-praise. Too often we rely on others for praise rather than giving it to ourselves. If you can become more reliant on yourself, you will be able to control your moods better, and you will avoid a lot of unnecessary disappointment. Controlling one's mood is one's *own* responsibility, not someone else's. Many relationship problems begin with the expectancy that the other person is responsible for your mood. Ultimately, this is an unfair demand to place on a loved one. Most bad moods are brought on by people talking themselves into them with too much self-criticism and too little self-praise. However, if you learn self-praise well, you can learn to take appropriate responsibility for your own moods.

Learning to stop engaging in useless self-criticism is every bit as important as learning to self-praise. When you catch yourself doing this, say to yourself: 'Stop criticising.' Then immediately switch to a self-praise thought. This thought-stopping technique is a proven and effective technique, but it *must* be practised. Since you are probably quite good at criticising yourself, you may need hundreds of practice trials of thought-stopping and thought-switching to break this habit. It probably took thousands, or more likely millions, of trials for you to learn the habit so well, and so a few hundred practices to change things isn't so bad. If you are really a 'pro', your negative, self-defeating thoughts may be almost automatic. This means you will have to pay special attention to catch them. Often they are such a part of you that unless you concentrate, you may not recognize them as they fly by.

Thought-stopping and thought-switching can be hard to do initially, but the more you practise the better you will get at it. If you practise enough, it will eventually become a habit itself. And this is a goal worth striving for, since it leads to a more positive view of yourself and an end to those negative thoughts which precipitate depression. Even if you feel silly at first, keep at it. Before long it will pay off.

Minimizing Unpleasant Experiences

Another factor which contributes to depression is continually having to face aversive situations. Unavoidably, all of us experience many unpleasant events. However, there are ways to see that one is placed in uncomfortable situations less often and ways to minimize the importance of them when they can't be avoided.

Controlling Chronic Pain

Those who are depressed or in chronic pain tend to evaluate experiences as more aversive. They also tend to dwell upon experiences evaluated as aversive relatively more than they think about those evaluated as positive. Since the quality of events (pleasant, neutral or aversive) is largely an *evaluative* judgment, how often and in what way we think about them can, in fact, be controlled by the same techniques just mentioned—thought-stopping and thought-switching. Focussing all of one's thoughts on anticipated or past unpleasant events is just as needless and destructive as dwelling on one's negative attributes. Moreover, such mis-directed attention always blows things out of all proportion. When you catch yourself imagining catastrophes, major or minor, stop and refocus your thoughts on something else. Of course it takes practice, but you can do it if you start conscientiously working on it.

The other way to minimize aversive experiences is to actually eliminate the sources of unpleasantness in circum-stances that you now find uncomfortable. To do this you must first analyse exactly what it is that is making specific events aversive for you. What makes people feel negative about any given situation is a very individual thing, but there are some general problems that you may find will help you define sources of unpleasantness:

1. Social anxiety: fear that you will say or do the 'wrong' thing; fear that others will not find you interesting; not knowing what to do in a given situation.
2. Excessive self-criticism: having rigid, unrealistic standards for yourself; reviewing and criticising yourself when you don't perform the way you think you should *always* perform.
3. Lack of assertiveness: allowing others to walk all over you; not standing up for your rights and feeling bad about it later.
4. Over-aggressiveness: infringing on other people's rights to keep them from infringing on yours.

By recognizing them, facing them head-on as problems and

learning the necessary skills to overcome them, you can eliminate such sources of unpleasantness. Learning to be more socially confident, more appropriately assertive or learning to turn off self-criticism and turn on self-praise often can alter many aversive situations into neutral or even pleasant ones. Chapter 11, 'Recognizing and Solving Other Problems Which May Aggravate Pain', discusses ways to deal with these problems in more detail.

Sometimes there are problems which cause us to feel negative or anxious, but which are not really *our* problems. Of course, we cannot hope to solve everybody else's problems for them. So long as we are not actually *causing* someone else's problem, it is not really our responsibility. Ultimately, each person is responsible for himself. Unfortunately though, people will often abandon their responsibility for their own problems and try to unload them on you. If this happens, you have four basic choices:

1. You can assert your rights and ask that they be respected. After all, it is simply not fair for you to be burdened with someone else's responsibilities when you have enough of your own.
2. You can attempt to persuade the other person that they should seek professional help for the problem. That's what therapeutic agencies are for.
3. You can choose simply to disregard the effects of the other person's problem on you by evaluating it as not important.
4. You can avoid contact whenever possible with the person who is the source of the problem.

Of course the first three of the above choices are the better ones and should be tried first. If they fail, however, the fourth choice may be effective in demonstrating to the other person that problem behaviour does not elicit your attention and leads you to avoid him instead. Since most people like attention and since most problem behaviour is maintained by attention (even scolding or arguing can be attention), withdrawal of attention can serve to lessen the frequency of the problem behaviour.

The other person learns that this is not the right way to get your attention. Additionally, of course, the fourth method does remove you from the aversive situation so that you can concentrate on getting on with your own life.

Maximizing Pleasant Experiences

Maximizing pleasure and joy in your life is really much easier than you probably imagine it to be. There are several simple things you can do about it. The most obvious one is to *do* more enjoyable things. Most often this is a matter that is completely under your control. All it requires is that you give some thought to what you find truly enjoyable and then schedule it more often. You can also learn to get more out of pleasant activities by focussing more on the enjoyment. There are, in fact, three types of potential enjoyment — anticipatory (looking forward to something), the here-and-now (enjoyment as the event takes place) and retrospection (memory of the pleasant experience). Each of these can and should be used to the fullest.

Let's begin with recognizing and scheduling more enjoyable activities. People who are depressed often balk at this suggestion. 'Nothing,' they maintain, 'is pleasurable anymore.' Of course, that is true only if you make it that way. But even if you're not willing to admit that activities are actually enjoyable, there are still some activities you prefer to do over others. If necessary, begin with those.

Sit down with your partner now and make up a list of things you enjoy doing. They can be things that you do by yourself or with friends. Suggestions for some activity categories to start you thinking are given on pages 99-101. Some of the items may be important or special things (e.g. going to lunch with a friend, taking a class in astronomy or weaving, reading a new book), but others may be small things that you do every day anyway (e.g. having a cup of coffee, taking a hot bath or shower, watching the television news). Part of this exercise is to help you focus on the pleasure of even the activities that you have come to treat perfunctorily. That is why it's important to list all the things you find pleasant, even those you do anyway. Once you have written down everything you and your partner can think of, place the list somewhere prominent, as you do with your contracts and graphs.

Suggested Pleasant Activities

Below is a list of types of activities that many people find enjoyable. A few examples are given to start you thinking. Underline examples that appeal to you, then add your own ideas in the space provided.

1. Self-care activities: having my hair done, trimming my beard, taking a hot shower, painting my fingernails, getting dressed up,

_____

_____   _____

_____

2. Food and where you like eating it: chicken at Colonel Sanders, homemade biscuits in front of the TV, steak at the local pub,

_____

_____

_____

3. Drinks and where you like drinking them: soft drink at the milkbar, beer at the local pub, wine at the wine bar, hot chocolate in bed,

_____

_____

_____

4. Recreational activities: going to a football match, playing golf, playing football or cricket with the kids, taking a country drive,

_____

_____

_____

5. Interpersonal activities: having friends over for dinner, talking on the phone to a friend, playing cards, going to a party, having sex with my partner,

_____

_____

_____

6. Mass media activities: going to a movie, watching news or sports on TV, reading the comics in the newspaper, listening to rock music on the radio,

_____

_____

_____

7. Appreciation activities: going to a concert, looking at art books, window shopping for cars, looking at fashion magazines, going to a museum,

_____

_____

_____

8. Educational activities: taking a class, reading a 'how to do it' book, watching educational programmes on TV, learning a new skill,

_____

_____

_____

9. Quiet activities: embroidery, putting together a puzzle, reading a novel,

_____

_____

_____

10. Creative activities: building a bookcase, making jewellery, painting, writing poetry, making up a new recipe,

_____

_____

_____

11. Travel activities: going for a weekend in the country, taking a coach 'joy ride', visiting historical or scenic landmarks,

_____

_____

_____

12. Searching activities: antique shopping, going to auctions or garage sales, bargain hunting, coin collecting, _____

_____

_____

_____

_____

Example Weekly Pleasant Activities List

This week I will try to do at least _____5_____ activities on the following list, marking a tick by each as I do it to keep track.

---

1. Sit and listen to my favourite record ✓ (Mon)

2. Give myself a manicure

3. Enjoy a piece of chocolate cake ✓ (Wed)

4. Sunbathe for 1 hour

5. Go out to 'Joe's' and have my favourite dish

6. Take a drive in the country ✓ (Sat)

7. Get dressed up ✓ (Fri)

8. Go out with Ken, Bill and Ruth

9. Read a magazine ✓ (Wed)

10. Stay up and watch the late night movie

11. Go on a shopping spree

12. Attend a concert

13. Spend all Saturday morning reading the paper

14. Write a poem on anything

15. Have a snuggle with Ken ✓ (Thur)

I feel proud of myself for meeting my goal to engage in pleasant activities! I will reward myself with self-praise and a bonus reward of

A new scarf to match my new coat

Weekly Pleasant Activities List

This week I will try to do at least _____ activities on the following list, marking a tick by each as I do it to keep track.

_____

1. _____

2. _____

3. _____

4. _____

5. _____

6. _____

7. _____

8. _____

9. _____

10. _____

11. _____

12. _____

13. _____

14. _____

15. _____

I feel proud of myself for meeting my goal to engage in pleasant activities! I will reward myself with self-praise and a bonus reward of

_____

Plan to do a certain number of activities from your list each week no matter how you feel. Page 102 shows a sample list of pleasant activities with a weekly goal at the top. Cross off activities as you do them. Then, at the end of the week, count up the number of activities you actually did to see whether you made your goal. Choose another of the activities on the list as a reward and self-reward yourself if you met your goal. Also remember to give yourself some praise.

Don't just wait for pleasant activities to come up. Think about them ahead of time. After all, anticipating something pleasant is part of the enjoyment. If, for example, you are vacuuming the living room and plan to sit down and have a cup of coffee when you have done a given amount, think about how good the coffee will taste. Imagine sitting in a nice, comfortable chair with your legs up. Think about what music you will put on the record player while you drink your coffee.

Next, don't let the pleasant events themselves go by without fully appreciating them. When you are sitting there drinking your coffee, savour each mouthful. Notice the lovely aroma. Feel the warmth spreading through your stomach. Listen to the music. Enjoy the melody or the rhythm. Think about how relaxed your body feels. Allow your thoughts to concentrate on these things. Do *not* worry about what you have to do next, what you're going to have for dinner, whether the kids will be home from school in time to get their homework done, what the doctor will say when you see him next, or anything else. Concentrate only on the pleasure of the moment. It is unfortunate to miss the pleasure in an activity by ignoring it, but it is worse yet to destroy it by thinking negative, anxious thoughts. Train your senses to enjoy by shutting off the negative, anxious thoughts—at least during pleasurable activities. Negative or anxious thoughts never solve anything anyway.

A technique which many people have found useful in trying to learn to exclude negative, unproductive thinking and to replace it with concentration on pleasure is to actually *schedule* worrying. If you find you *must* worry or have periods of feeling negative about yourself, schedule a specific time (for example a certain hour each day) to do it. Then, every time it crops up outside the scheduled hour, put the negative thought aside until the worry hour. Then, and only at the appointed hour, worry your heart out. But don't go beyond the end of your scheduled time slot.

Finally, in addition to thinking about pleasant activities ahead of time and getting the most out of them while doing them, think back afterwards on how enjoyable they were. You may even want to try describing activities to someone, perhaps when you are talking about your day. It's one way to recall and enjoy again something pleasant. But whether through describing them or just reviewing enjoyable activities in your mind, try to recall as many of the details as possible. Focusing on all the senses, try to conjure up specific images (the aroma of the coffee, the taste, the sound of the music, and the relaxed sensation in your body). Remembering a pleasant activity increases the enjoyment you get from anticipating the next repetition of that same activity, and so it comes full circle.

Since most people forget to focus on and enjoy the potentially pleasurable activities they already engage in, let's take another example to make the point clearer. Take a nice shower or bath, for instance. Hot showers or baths *can* be very enjoyable. It can be great to have a shower or bath in the late afternoon or evening especially after a hard day. They can also be very relaxing just before bedtime.

Let's imagine that you are driving home from work in rush hour traffic and you're thinking about an unpleasant conversation you've had with your boss. That stack of work you left unfinished on your desk is bothering you as well. Okay, now turn those thoughts off and think instead of the nice hot shower or bath you're going to have when you get home. Imagine taking off your work clothes and stepping into a nice hot tub of water, sinking back, and feeling the sensation of warmth and well-being. Now just relax, imagine the warmth. If you keep thinking about this instead of the traffic or the problems at work, you'll be in a much better frame of mind to

105

unwind and enjoy the evening.

Once you arrive home, explain to your partner that you'll be in a better mood for the rest of the evening if you take a nice relaxing bath or shower first. Few partners can resist the temptation of having you in a good mood. If you think that he or she may resent it, suggest that if you have a bath or shower first and relax, you'll do the dishes, help the children with homework, work out holiday plans, fix the latch on the door, or whatever.

If you want to enhance your enjoyment, appeal to more senses. Some of the enjoyment from simple things can come by elaborating them. For example, use bubble bath or bath oil (men can use these too). Take a drink or snack into the bath with you. Put some music on to listen to while bathing or provide it yourself by singing. Take a book or magazine in to read while in the bath (it may get a little wet, but, oh well). Have your partner come in and talk to you.

Remember to notice pleasurable sensations. Focus on them. Take your time. And praise yourself. Say that you deserve to relax. Do *not* think about work. Do *not* think about pain. But do have fun. Splash some water about. Baths and showers can be good play times, and adults need play as much as children. Feel the sleepy, content feeling come over you. Finally, take your time drying off. There should be no need to hurry. Put on something comfortable and maybe some pleasant fragrance.

If you really follow through with this approach to pleasurable activities you will find you are indeed in a better frame of mind. You will be more tolerant with your partner and children and enjoy the evening more.

The next day at work when things are getting to you, think back to your nice relaxing time in the bath, feel the hot water relaxing you, or think ahead to tonight.

A shower the next morning can be just as much fun in a different way. It can wake you up. It can be bracing. Splash. Enjoy it. Sing a little. Let the water pour on your face. Focus on the smell of soap or shampoo. Don't think about the day ahead. There will be time enough for that later. Enjoy your shower.

You will notice that there were several procedures employed in the above discussion which you should follow in your programme:

1. *Schedule* pleasant activities frequently (perhaps more frequently than you might ordinarily do them). Pleasant activities can be planned to follow a difficult task, as a reward.
2. *Focus* in on the *pleasure* (ahead of time, during and after the activity).
3. *Elaborate* the activity to include as many enjoyable things and as many senses as possible (sight, hearing, taste, touch and smell).
4. *Exclude* negative or anxious thoughts.
5. *Vary* the activity so that it doesn't get boring.
6. *Add self-praise* to the activity when it is used as a reward.

Maximizing Mastery Over the Environment

In addition to engaging in pleasurable activities, it is important to engage in activities which require mastery and thus can provide a sense of satisfaction or accomplishment. Some pleasurable activities may give us that feeling; others may not. Chapter 5, 'How to Resume More Normal Activity', provides you with a method of tackling problems of mastery. What this chapter does not address, however, is what *you* consider an accomplishment to be. Different people have vastly different criteria for what they consider accomplishment. When someone is not working on what he truly considers to be an accomplishment but instead on what others consider worthwhile, he may run into trouble. When you are only doing what others think you should do in order to meet with their approval, your goals may seem less important to you and, moreover, you may be excluding work on activities that *you* think you should do. This can also become a source of difficulty with self-praise. If you don't *really* consider what you are doing as praiseworthy, it may be hard to praise yourself genuinely. In this case, mastery and the sense of

Developing Life Goals

Six-month Goals	One-year Goals	Five-year Goals

accomplishment which accompanies it can become very elusive. This issue is discussed in more detail in Chapter 11 under the section titled 'Failure to Live Up to Expectations'.

In addition, problems with mastery can come from unrealistic expectations. If your goals are set too high, for example, mastery will remain out of reach. Or you may not have broken your goals into small enough steps (see Chapter 5). You must set realistic goals for yourself—goals at which you *can* succeed. Much of this book is aimed at establishing just that sort of pattern—setting goals, working on small enough units to gain success, even at big, seemingly impossible goals.

It may be, however, that activity goals such as walking, sitting, more recreational activities or controlling your pain medication do not seem important enough to *you*. Sometimes more long term or lofty goals are needed to help motivate oneself. If you think this is true for you, you may find it helpful to establish some of these goals for yourself as well. Spend some time working on the worksheet on page 108. Work out some goals for six months from now, one year from now, and five years from now. Each set of goals will work best if it works toward the next set. But remember that all goals, however big or small, should be worked on *gradually*, a little at a time. You may want to refer back to Chapter 5 to remind yourself how to break goals into task steps with target dates. Learning to set *realistic* goals, and programme rewards and rests are some of the more difficult but profitable skills to be acquired. Without these skills you will surely not succeed.

Summary

You *can* control your environment to make it give you more pleasurable experiences and less aversive ones. To do this you need to schedule pleasurable experiences, anticipate them, get maximum enjoyment from them when they are taking place and remember them frequently afterwards. Thought-stopping and thought-switching can be practised to turn off negative, anxious thoughts. Scheduling worry times works to limit mental time spent on negative thoughts. Expanding the mental time spent on thinking about pleasure is important.

Recognizing and working toward solving problem behaviours that get us into trouble can give us a sense of control. Recognizing that we are not responsible for other people's problems and not falling into the trap of taking on the responsibilities of others can help minimize aversive experiences.

Most important is self-praise and self-reinforcement. Recognizing oneself as a good, capable, attractive person is important. If you can't do this, you need practice. Working on noticing and appreciating your own assets (never mind your faults; you've been focusing on them long enough) will work toward your liking yourself better and an improved mood state. All these things will help you to fight off the depression of chronic pain.

If depression continues to be a special problem for you despite the suggestions here, you may find it helpful to consult a self-help book written solely for the problem of depression, such as *Control Your Depression,* a paperback book by Peter Lewinsholn, Richardo Munoz, Mary Ann Youngren and Antonette Zeiss. For more information see the 'Further Reading' section on pages 190-202. Or you may wish to seek professional help as suggested earlier in the chapter on page 90.

7.   Controlling the Pain Killers

George, the school teacher introduced on page 10 who was taking too much codeine, was prescribed a 'pain cocktail' equivalent in strength to his former level of medication. Gradually, over a 16-week period, the codeine which he had taken for six years was reduced with small decreases taking place every few days. Because his medication problem had been severe, his pain cocktail was initially taken every four hours under medical supervision. However, he soon did so well that the pain cocktail was turned over to him to administer to himself. He was rigorous about taking his cocktail on the prescribed time schedule. When he went out, he would estimate how long he planned to be gone and take the right amount of pain cocktail in a small jar in his pocket.

The irritability and tiredness which he had previously shown began to disappear as his medication was reduced and as he became physically stronger. He began taking much more pride in how he looked; in fact the contrast was so great that people who had not seen him for a few weeks did not recognize him. Being able to work himself off his codeine helped his self-confidence, which had been at an all-time low. His pain became so reduced that he decided to enrol in classes to train as a real estate salesman. He enjoyed this activity and later passed his real estate licence examination with flying colours. His wife, also a school teacher, was delighted. She reported that before George began the pain cocktail, the family had been at the end of its rope.

This chapter pertains to you if your use of analgesic medication is chronic (extending over a time span of more than a few months) or bothers you, anyone in your family, or your doctor. 'Analgesic' refers to pain-killing medication. Often people take several kinds of medication for different problems and don't know which one is for which problem. It is very important for you to find out, at least, which of your medications are analgesics and which are not. *In this chapter we are discussing only pain medication or medication taken to control pain, not other types of medication.*

It is best if you work on controlling your medication with your doctor's help. If he is willing, it is a good idea to have him read this chapter, as well as the section on the 'Medication Trap' in Chapter 2. You may wish to re-read that section yourself before reading on.

Your first step toward controlling your pain killers is to make a list of your medications, their purposes, the dosage of each, and how frequently you think you take each—on average days and on bad days. A sample layout for an **Estimated Medication Record** is given on page 113. The name, potency and recommended dosage of your medication can usually be found on the front or side of the bottle. Potency, of course, refers to the amount of active drug in each tablet. If you do not know or are not sure of the purpose of a medication, leave the purpose space blank and take your chart in to ask the doctor who prescribed it. When estimating how many pills you take of each medicine on an average day and on a bad day, try to be as accurate as you can. Typically, people tend to *underestimate* their usage, often because they are simply unaware of their habits.

If more than one doctor is prescribing medication for you, take your chart to each doctor who prescribed it. In this way you will be assured that each doctor knows what you are getting from the other. Some drugs do not mix well and it is of great importance that each of your doctors is fully aware of all the medication you take.

Estimated Medication Record

List *all* the medications you take. If you co not know the purpose of your medication, your doctor will be able to help you fill out this column. The potency of your medication will be noted on the pill bottle. In the last two columns, estimate your medication usage on an average day and on a bad day.

Name of Medication	Purpose	Potency of dosage	Average day's usage	Bad day's usage
1.				
2.				
3.				
4.				
5.				
6.				
7.				
8.				
9.				
10.				

But it is also important for *you* to know what you are taking and what it is for. Often doctors are so busy that they don't explain your medication to you fully. However, you have the right to ask questions and to know the whys and wherefores of your doctors' prescriptions. After all, it is your body which is receiving the drugs you take.

You should be able to get satisfaction from asking your doctor. If you have trouble finding this information, either you are not being assertive enough, or your doctor is one of the very few who doesn't think patients should know such things. But generally the problem will be that you are being unassertive. The best way to ask your doctor is by showing him your chart and saying that you would like his help in filling in the purpose spaces. There are, of course, several professional books available which can give you the needed information. Most libraries or pharmacists will have a copy of *MIMS* or a dictionary of drugs in which you can find information on the ingredients, general purpose, usual dosage and side effects of the medication(s) you are using.

Once you know the names, purposes and effects of your medication(s), you will be ready to begin working on actually controlling your intake of analgesics or pain killers. As mentioned above, the process is best done with your doctor's help, knowledge and assistance.

As you will remember from the section on the Medication Trap, analgesics were made to be taken for acute, short-term pain. There are two major problems with the *chronic use* of pain killers:

1. Over time the body develops a greater and greater tolerance for the drug so that more and more is needed, until finally even large amounts have little or no effect on the pain.
2. Medication taken irregularly, only when pain is at its worst, actually reinforces the pain response, and over time, gradually makes the pain episodes worse. Thus, not only do analgesics lose their effectiveness over time, but they may eventually *aggravate* pain, while increasing the likelihood of side effects.

Most chronic pain patients actually realize that they are no longer getting much benefit from their analgesics, but because they are still under the belief that they *should* be getting benefit (the pervasiveness of the 'pills cure everything' myth) and the fact that the doctor is still prescribing them (which he may be doing simply because you are asking for them), they keep taking them in larger and larger dosages. As mentioned in the section in Chapter 2 on the Medication Trap, the problem of medication aggravating pain is a subtle one. Over time, a relationship is established between your pain and the taking of medication. With hundreds, even thousands of repetitions of this connection, your body may *learn* to actually hurt more. If your pain has gradually been getting worse over the years, this may, in fact, be one of the causes. You have been *reinforcing* your pain with medication.

The next step is for you to keep a **Medication Diary** that will allow you to determine exactly how much medication you take and when you take it. You should have already filled out your own **Estimated Medication Record**. The **Estimated Medication Record** represents what you *think* you take. The **Medication Diary**, by contrast, will be a record of what you actually *do* take. It should be interesting to see whether your estimates are correct. Note that the **Medication Diary**, which is shown on pages 116-7, asks you to record your level of pain, a well as the name and dosage of medication. Before proceeding further, keep your **Medication Diary** for one week.

Once you have completed your **Medication Diary** for one week, you are ready to analyse it by answering the following questions:

1. Did you take your pain medication at regular or irregular intervals?
2. Did you try to resist taking medication until the pain was really quite bad?
3. Did you take more on bad days and less on good days (consult your pain rating scale)?
4. At what pain rating level did you usually take medication?

Medication Diary

Record the type and amount of pain medication each time you take
something. Also record your average pain level for each waking hour
throughout the day.

	Time	Pain Medication	Amount	Pain Level: 0-10*
a.m.	6-7.00			
	7-8.00			
	8-9.00			
	9-10.00			
	10-11.00			
	11-12.00			
p.m.	12-1.00			
	1-2.00			
	2-3.00			
	3-4.00			
	4-5.00			
	5-6.00			
	6-7.00			
	7-8.00			
	8-9.00			

	9–10.00			
	10–11.00			
	11–12.00			
a.m.	12–1.00			
	1–2.00			
	2–3.00			
	3–4.00			
	4–5.00			
	5–6.00			

*Pain level: 0 = no pain   10 = severe pain.

5. Was there a pattern to your high pain level or greater medication usage (e.g. was it worse at a certain time of the day)?
6. If there was an identifiable pattern, can you relate it to any environmental event(s) (e.g. being alone, driving home from work, etc.)?

If you answered as most pain patients do, that you take pain medication on an irregular schedule, that you try to resist taking it, and that you take more on bad days than on good days or when the pain rating level is fairly high, then it is very likely that your medication habits have in the long run been making your pain problem worse, not better.

The first thing to remember about pain medication is that it is meant to be taken *regularly* on a *set time schedule*. It works best that way, and it also is thereby dissociated from your pain episodes.

The next important thing to be aware of is that large dosages of pain killers are very hard on your liver and kidneys, which have to process all drugs. Since you are probably getting very little pain relief from it anyway, it would almost certainly be a good idea for you to cut down on, or eventually cut out, pain medication altogether.

If you decide to make cutting down or getting off pain medication your goal, it should be done *gradually*. Getting off medication, whether the addictive type or not, has the best chance of working if it's done *slowly*. Patients (and doctors) sometimes try to stop medication all at once. This is a bit like trying a starvation diet. It is both dangerous and unlikely to succeed. It generally ends up a failure, resulting in dependence or fear of dependence on the medication becoming stronger than ever. Getting patients' analgesics under control is part of the programme at many Pain Clinics, but the process is always done gradually and systematically.

If you have now accepted that your chronic pain is something with which you will have to live, and you are no longer seeking a cure, then you do not want to take pain medication forever. Besides reinforcing the pain, having little effectiveness for relief and causing stress on liver and kidneys as explained above, it serves to remind you, your family and others that you are a 'sick' person. The aim of this book is to have you behave like, be seen as and feel like a 'well' person.

A proven technique for systematically reducing your pain medication involves the use of a 'pain cocktail'. The pain cocktail is something your chemist can mix up at your doctor's order. It involves mixing your medication in a masking agent such as cherry syrup. The masking agent ensures that each time you take your medication it will appear the same, no matter what dosages are contained within it. (See the diagram on page 119.) This makes the reduction process easier, as will be explained below. To put the pain cocktail plan to work the following steps are necessary:

How to Use the Pain Cocktail

Step 1: Mix active ingredients into masking agent

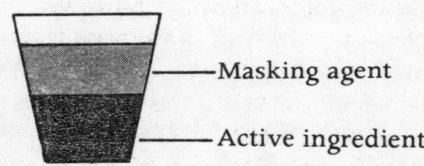

—Masking agent

—Active ingredient

Step 2: Give pain cocktail on a *regular* schedule, e.g. 4 hourly

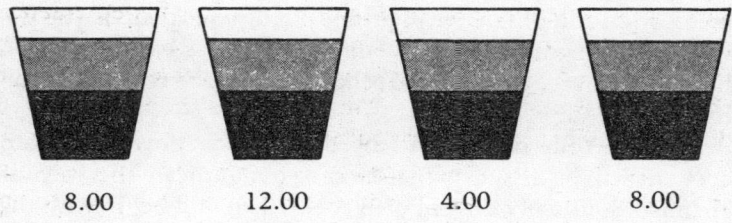

8.00   12.00   4.00   8.00

Step 3: Fade active ingredients *slowly*

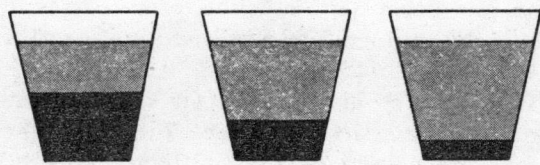

Step 4: Extend or fade time schedule, e.g. 6 hourly, then 8 hourly, etc.

8.00   2.00   8.00   etc.

Controlling Chronic Pain

Step 1: From your **Medication Diary,** you and your doctor should determine an optimum time schedule at which you should take medication. Note how far apart you have usually been taking it and time your new schedule initially with intervals a little shorter than the average of your old ones. This will help you get in the habit of taking the medication *before* you hurt badly. The time schedule should be a *perfectly regular* one, such as every three hours, every four hours, every five hours, every six hours. Do not try to set yourself a difficult goal here. The idea is to *succeed* in establishing a regular schedule for your medication usage. For example if you decide on every four hours, and you generally take your first pills at 7.30 a.m., you might wish to make your schedule: 7.30 a.m., 11.30 a.m., 3.30 p.m., 7.30 p.m., 11.30 p.m. If you don't usually take pain medication at night, leave nightime out of your plan. If you do, work out a regular time for your night dose as well. Once you have determined such a time schedule, you are ready to go on to the next step.

Step 2: Your doctor will need to decide how your pain cocktail will be mixed so that he can communicate this to your chemist. Your daily dose of pain cocktail should begin with the average amount of analgesic you have been taking, or even slightly more, so that you can ease into this routine with no discomfort. He will have to work out how much of each pain medication you will receive at each time interval. It is advisable for doctors and chemists to mix the formula so that patients take 10 cc (including medication *and* masking agent) of the pain cocktail each time.

Step 3: Step three involves getting rid of all other pain medication you have in the house. This strengthens your commitment and helps you to avoid temptation. It also is a good gesture or sign to yourself that you are really serious about reducing your intake of drugs. Get rid of all the old medication by flushing it down the toilet.

Step 4: Once the schedule for the pain cocktail has been worked out, complete the **Pain Cocktail Contract** found on page 121. Note the planned times to take the pain cocktail

Pain Cocktail Contract

I hereby agree to adhere strictly to the schedule below in taking my pain cocktail. I also agree not to take the pain cocktail or any other pain medication at other times. (For each day of the week, tick whether you took your cocktail on schedule.)

Time Schedule	Day 1	Day 2	Day 3	Day 4	Day 5	Day 6	Day 7

For complete success in meeting my pain cocktail schedule, I will reward myself with

_____

_____

Signed

_____

Date

down the left-hand column. After it is filled in, place the contract next to the pain cocktail bottle. Over the next weeks, mark on the contract each time you take the cocktail on time. Also choose a fairly significant reward that you can give yourself at the end of every week in which you are a complete success—dinner at a favourite restaurant, a new book or record, a new article of clothing, play or concert tickets, a Sunday drive, a new tool or household item, or something else that will help motivate you. Then be sure to give yourself the reward as soon as possible after the conclusion of a successful week.

Step 5: Now you are ready to begin your pain cocktail. The time schedule you worked out must be *strictly adhered to*. The pain cocktail is to be taken on time, even if you don't have any pain at all. Also, neither it nor any other pain killing medication is to be taken between scheduled intervals—even if your pain is really bad. It is important that you retrain your body so that pain medication is no longer given when it signals pain. The new system means pain medication on a *schedule*. If you plan to go out, pour the amount you should take into a smaller bottle, put it in your handbag, briefcase, pocket, or in the glove box of your car. At the appropriate time, slip away to the toilet and take your cocktail on schedule. It can usually be done very unobtrusively.

Step 6: Once you have become accustomed to a regular pain cocktail schedule you may wish to make an agreement with your doctor to *gradually*, over a given time period, reduce the amount of pain medication in it. It is advisable for you to choose an end goal with your doctor, such as 'go off pain killers completely' or 'cut my use of pain killers in half' over an agreed time period—for example three months, six months, or longer. A new prescription can then be mixed each week, or every two weeks, at which time the amount of medication may be slightly reduced. It is nearly always best if you don't know the exact details—the exact timing or size of reductions in the prescription. This may sound like a contradiction of what was said earlier about knowing what you are taking, but in fact, you *will* know what is in the pain cocktail as the beginning and the end goal will be set by you. The rationale for not knowing the details of the small reductions is to prevent one's body and mind responding to this knowledge by causing undue pain attacks related to known medication changes. In the area of pain, there has been a great deal of scientific research which shows unequivocally that the mind is particularly susceptible to suggestions and expectation. In other words, expectations have a big influence over the pain perceptions of even the most stoic among us. So, we can be responsible for the general plan of regular scheduling and gradual reduction, but it is really better not to be aware of the details. Let the doctor and chemist do that. But be sure to do your part during the programme by continuing to make weekly contracts with yourself and by using weekly rewards. If you find yourself failing, try increasing the strength of your rewards or go to daily rewards, as explained in the chapter on exercise programmes, Chapter 5.

Step 7: If your goal is to go off pain medication entirely, as you get close to the end of your programme your pain cocktail will have only a small amount of pain killer left in it. At this point, you and your doctor may decide to finish the programme more quickly by spacing out the intervals in your schedule. For example, if you were on a four-hourly schedule you could go to a six-hourly schedule, and after a couple of weeks, to an eight-hourly schedule, then a twelve-hourly schedule. Finally you could reduce to one cocktail every other day and then no more when you are ready. But this altering of your schedule should only be done toward the end of your programme, and only under the supervision of your doctor.

Step 8: If your goal, however, has been only to reduce your pain medication to some fraction of your former intake, you can switch back to pills when you have reached your goal. But the time schedule should remain *strictly* in force, with no skipping of pills or extra pills taken. If at some later time you should decide to cut down further, you can return to the pain cocktail and use the same procedure again.

123

Controlling Chronic Pain

The pain cocktail can also be used for other over-used or abused medication such as sleeping tablets or tranquillizers. The above section is restricted to pain medication, but if you and your doctor decide that other medication, such as those just mentioned, should go into the cocktail, this can be done. Or separate cocktails can be formulated for other problem drugs. Sleep Cocktails or Nerve Cocktails can be equally effective means of weaning patients from medication habits which are hard or dangerous to break suddenly.

There may be some cases in which it is impossible for you to use the pain cocktail. You may, for instance, find it hard to convince either your doctor or your chemist to prescribe or prepare the cocktail, although most are willing. However, if this is the case, it may be possible to apply the principles of the pain cocktail to pill-taking. The primary advantages of the cocktail over the use of pills are:

1. Pills often come in fairly large, set amounts so that it is hard to work out the gradual programme of small reductions which can be changed easily and reliably in the pain cocktail. Typically, pills can only be broken into a few pieces, and the pieces may not always be equal. (Breaking up tablets also frequently makes them taste worse.)

2. With pills you will unavoidably always have to be fully aware of your exact dosages and of every little change in your intake. This gives your body and mind a chance to *expect* difficulty when the dosages are reduced, and this makes it far more likely that trouble will arise.

Nevertheless, if your doctor or chemist insists on the use of pill reduction, the method can still work to reduce your pain killers. The main idea is to put your medication-taking on a set *time schedule,* and when you decide to reduce the overall dosage, to do so *gradually* in *small* amounts over a fairly long time span. You must, of course, work out the amounts of reduction and the exact dates *ahead of time,* and then rigorously stick to this plan. It is a bad idea to start making changes in your programme based on how you *feel,* and with pills, there can be a greater temptation. If you do stray from your plan, you will soon find yourself back at the beginning, with your pain levels controlling your medication usage. The aim of this programme is to break the learned connection between how you feel (i.e. your pain) and your medication habits.

If your pain medication is taken by injection, it can be converted to an oral form and the pain cocktail used. Continuous injections for the rest of your life are, of course, an even worse idea than continuous pill taking. If you have been taking pain medication by injection, change to oral medication can sometimes be difficult to do in a self-help programme. If you are receiving regular (or irregular) injections of pain killers, you may want to go to a Pain Clinic or undergo a period of hospitalization in order to work yourself off this type of analgesic administration.

One final note: The pain cocktail procedure, of course, is advisable only if you have *chronic* pain and *chronic* pain medication usage. Such a procedure would not be advisable for the occasional pain episode, such as the occasional headache, and the subsequent pain killer you may take at that time. On the other hand, if you have continual headaches (or other types of chronic pain) and if you continually use pain killers, then this procedure is advisable.

Use of the pain cocktail to regularize and slowly reduce your pain medication makes the process as easy as possible. However, you are on a retraining programme and you may find that your body has some difficulty adjusting to your new plans for it. After all, you may be changing or breaking years of habit. This is why it is important to remember that the steps are made small enough to ensure success. Above all, remember that if you are strict with yourself in adhering to the prescribed regimen, your pain episodes will soon be under much better control and your body *will* learn a more stable, regular pattern, often leading to reduced pain sensations.

8. What to Do and What Not to Do When You Are in Pain

There are many ways to cope with pain. Coping with pain means reducing the importance of pain in your life, and this usually involves learning new ways of responding, behaving, talking or thinking, which diminish pain and increase the importance of other aspects of your life. It also involves learning *not* to engage in certain behaviours, topics of conversation or thoughts which may seem natural but which tend to make the pain worse, increase its importance and take up your energies to the exclusion of other things. This chapter will suggest ways that you can behave, talk and think which will, *with enough practice,* begin to diminish the importance of pain. Nothing happens overnight; the process is a slow one. You will need to practise the procedures regularly and repeatedly. But if you have come this far in the book, you have probably already accepted the idea that there are no instant answers and that no one can solve your chronic pain for you. You can, however, eventually learn to cope better with your pain.

As you will recall from Chapter 5, it is essential to be active rather than inactive and to make your life as normal as possible. You have to learn to stop thinking of yourself as a sick person.

It is also important that you are not seen as an invalid by other people. People respond to any signs that you are sick or in pain by placing you in the sick role. If you allow yourself to be treated as an invalid, before long you will be one. If, on the other hand, you can get others to treat you as a well person, before long you will feel better and less in pain.

Many of the following suggestions are aimed at helping you to avoid the appearance of being sick so that you will not be slotted by others into the 'sick role'. These ideas can also help you to learn not to focus so much on pain and problems. In effect, this means you will be learning to resist giving in to the pain. Instead, by assuming a 'well role' (even when you do not feel good), you will gradually gain the upper hand with your pain—in fact, as well as in appearance. The following suggestions on how to assume a 'well role' are ones that have proved useful to many other pain patients. Study them and then try them for yourself:

1. Always, no matter how badly you feel, get completely dressed first thing in the morning. Do not continue to wear your bedclothes or dressing gown. If you are dressed for bed, others will respond to you as if you are an invalid. Moreover, getting dressed will help you avoid the temptation to return to bed during the day.

2. Avoid reclining during the day. This means resisting any urges to lie down on the couch, the bed or the floor, including periods during which you are reading, watching television or doing other activities. It can be difficult to change your habits if you have been used to taking frequent rests in a reclining position. You may have to wean yourself away from the habit gradually. Try reducing the amount of time you spend reclining by five or ten minutes per day. It may even be a good idea to make a contract with yourself similar to the ones explained in Chapter 5. Decide on gradually decreasing daily goals (minutes spent reclining) and on daily rewards. You can then keep a graph of your progress. If you have been working on your exercise programme (also described in

Chapter 5), you should be able to begin substituting other activities—walking or sitting—for reclining ones. Within a few weeks you should have weaned yourself completely away from daytime reclining. Of course, once you have broken the habit, it is important not to give in and return to it, even on an occasional basis. In addition to worsening a pain problem, reclining during the day can aggravate the insomnia which often afflicts pain patients.

3. When you are in pain, engage in an activity and stay with it. Bake something, read something, play cards, make a list, take a walk, take a drive in the car, put a puzzle together, work on a hobby, or watch television. In other words, do something. Involve yourself in any activity other than thinking about, caring for or trying to relieve your pain. The important thing is to draw the focus of your mind and body away from the pain. This may be difficult at first, but it should become easier as you stay with the activity you have chosen. Force your mind and body to become involved and engrossed in that activity. It helps to keep a list of possible activities on hand which can be used as distractions whenever you need them. In Chapter 3 you and your partner made up a list of potential activities which you can now draw upon. Choose something from this list and get started.

4. Pamper yourself. Be nice to yourself. But don't do it by taking it easy. Go shopping and buy a new article of clothing. Go to the hairdresser, take extra care with your grooming, take a bubble bath, grow a moustache or beard or try shaving them off if you have them, buy a new perfume or aftershave lotion, get some new makeup or jewellery, or put on that favourite dress, jumper or shirt. (Looking better can substantially improve your outlook.) Give yourself any little special consideration, so long as it involves being active.

5. Do not act as though you are in pain. Try to get rid of any 'pain behaviours' which may indicate to others that you are feeling bad. Make an effort to walk normally, get out of

chairs normally, avoid rubbing sore areas, avoid wincing or looking drawn. Try smiling, winking, laughing, or looking relaxed and happy. Most people believe that how one feels affects how one behaves, but the reverse is equally true. How one behaves has a powerful influence on how one feels. If one acts as if he feels fine, he really will feel better. Try it; you will be surprised! Concentrating on this effort will also serve to distract your thoughts from the focus on pain.

6. Make regular plans to do things with other people—family or friends. And *never* change your plans or back out of a scheduled activity because you 'don't feel up to it'. Even if your pain seems bad, force yourself to honour scheduled or planned activities without letting others know you don't feel well. And, at all cost, do not give anybody the impression that you are being a martyr. If you don't feel well, just go along and keep it to yourself. Chances are that you will feel better as time passes. Of course, as discussed in Chapter 5, it is important to plan your activities so that they are well within your capabilities. As you become gradually stronger, you can plan more and more demanding activities. But the rate of increase should be carefully paced.

7. Setting up and sticking to a daily routine is a good idea. It is easier to do things if they are regularly scheduled and sequenced. Give some thought to the best ways to order your day. You may wish to follow more strenuous activities with more restful ones rather than having two strenuous ones in a row. Resting (sitting, not reclining) is not bad as long as you use it as a reward. Take a rest break *after completion* of some scheduled activity. Many patients, in fact, find it helpful to schedule their rest periods as well as their activities. Rest breaks can be a nice time to have a cup of coffee, read a book, magazine or newspaper, work on a puzzle, or knit. They can also provide a good time to practise the relaxation exercises which will be discussed later in Chapter 10.

8. You may be in the habit of making special requests to family members when you are in pain. For example, you may ask someone to bring you your medicine or your hot water bottle; you may ask a family member for a back rub; you may expect the house to be quiet or ask your spouse to keep the kids from fighting; you may want the television off or the stereo turned down; you may ask that your dinner be brought to you in bed rather than joining the family at the table. Whatever requests of this sort you have made in the past should in future be abolished. Avoid back or head rubs; join the family for dinner; don't make any special requests for peace and quiet. If you have carefully read Chapter 7, 'Controlling the Pain Killers', you will know that you should not be taking pain medication when you hurt, but according to a regular schedule. When the scheduled time arrives, get the pain cocktail yourself and take it quietly. Don't use special equipment or special rituals to 'ease' the pain. Get rid of any special equipment you have—hot water bottles, heating pads, hospital beds, hydroculators or special cushions. Avoid special rituals such as standing on one leg or sitting in a special position with legs raised or a pillow behind your head. While they may seem to work on a short term basis, all of these things only add to the long term problem of having your life cluttered up with pain-relief activities. Besides, having special equipment around reminds you and others that you are ill; in turn that means everybody is going to respond to you in that way.

9. If you have been maintaining an exercise programme as outlined in Chapter 5, you will gradually find yourself able to do more. You may be able to begin to do things that up until now others have been doing for you. Making this sort of change usually requires breaking established habits about who does what. And often it is just as hard for the other person as it is for you. The best way to break these habits is to begin doing these things for yourself on a small scale to demonstrate to the other person that you *can* do

them. This may involve such simple things as reaching things for yourself. Stop the other person from doing such things for you and do it in front of him successfully. Explain to him that your exercise programme is working. Part of the reconditioning process involves reconditioning other family members' expectations as well as your own.

10. Do not tell anyone about it when you are in pain. Keep your conversation on other topics. If someone asks you how you feel, tell a little white lie and say 'fine', then change the topic. Do not permit others to talk about you as a sick person. If they try, change the subject. By the same token, do not talk about yourself as an invalid. Avoid telling people about your treatments or the effects of having chronic pain. Above all, avoid discussing how you *feel*. Talk instead about what you have been *doing*. Talk about what *others* have been doing. Ask questions. Show interest in others. Chronic pain patients have a tendency to become somewhat self-centred. But people don't enjoy hearing you talk only about yourself. Give them a chance to discuss their interests and activities too.

11. What you *focus* your thoughts on will play a part in how you feel. Controlling your mental focus is a skill that you can learn. Focusing thoughts on pain or the hopelessness of your situation is what you most likely have been doing. But you can just as easily learn to focus your thoughts on more positive things. Compose a list of pleasant things that you can substitute for negative thoughts: your holiday next year, your work, your weekend plans, or something concerning your children or friends. You may wish to create pleasant scenes or images to bring to mind when you are resting or trying to fall asleep. Conjure up one or two pleasant scenes and then practise them. For example, you might imagine lying on a bright, sandy beach, feeling the warm sun beating down on your body, listening to the sound of the surf and smelling the salt spray and seaweed. Use as many of these senses as you can in describing the scene to yourself. Imagine the sights, sounds, smells, tastes

and feel of the situation. Practise your scene each time you are relaxing. Hold it in your mind and continue elaborating it.

12. Change your attitudes about pain. You have probably been emphasising your problem to yourself. Each of us talks to himself using what is called 'internal dialogue'. In their internal dialogue, pain patients often tell themselves how terrible and utterly hopeless their situation is and how totally inadequate they are to cope with it. Continually replaying such messages to yourself only serves to make your problem worse. Therefore, it is important that you try to change your internal dialogue in the direction of more constructive thoughts. Instead of saying: 'It is hopeless; my life is ruined', try saying to yourself such statements as: 'Chronic pain is not pleasant, but I can cope. By practising my new strategies, I will be able to cope with my pain and lead a more normal life. I'm in control here, not the pain.' Take some file cards and write a different coping statement on each one. Start with the ones above, then add some statements of your own. Practise them many times each day. Each time you catch yourself thinking of your pain, switch thoughts. Pull out your file cards and rehearse your coping statements. Try adding one coping statement to your collection each day.

13. Another technique known to psychologists as 'stress innoculation' may be of some help to you. This procedure requires you to use your imagination to practise coping with pain problems ahead of time. The practising is done while sitting comfortably in a chair with eyes closed. First, you bring to mind a potential problem and then you imagine yourself coping successfully with it. For example, you might imagine what you would do if you came down with a severe pain attack on the Saturday that the family has planned a picnic and country walk and you have promised to go along. Using the ideas discussed in this chapter, imagine not mentioning your pain to the family. Picture yourself driving the car, preparing the fire, playing

with the children, focusing on these activities instead of the pain. Rehearse the coping statements that you would say: 'I'm in control, not the pain. It will go away before long.' Now imagine the pain gradually fading away. Praise yourself for coping successfully.

This kind of rehearsal can help you cope more effectively by preparing you for situations. Try to anticipate problem areas and rehearse your coping procedures in your mind ahead of time. It will make the actal events go much more easily when they come up.

Summary

When you are in pain, it is very important that you do not give in to it. What you focus your attention and thoughts on will, to some extent, guide how you feel. Focusing on pain and pain-relief procedures tends to intensify your perception of pain. By contrast, focusing on other things will help to diminish pain. For this reason suggestions are made in this chapter for getting involved in absorbing activities and not allowing yourself to think or talk about pain or to engage in relief rituals. In addition to directing your focus away from pain, you should try to appear as normal and well as possible. Both you and those around you will be affected by how you act. If you act sick, your family and friends will place you in the 'sick role'. If you act well (even if, at first, you don't feel it), others will treat you more normally. This will cause you to respond more normally and eventually to *feel* more normal. None of this is easy to do. It will require practice. The next chapter will discuss how your family can help you.

9. How You, the Family, Can Help

Partners or families of chronic pain patients often feel as helpless as the patient. Over months, and sometimes years, they watch their loved one suffer pain, become progressively weaker and more inactive and grow demoralized and depressed as hoped for relief from treatment after treatment does not materialize. After years of having normal family functioning restricted, making special accommodations, and having the family focusing on one member's pain problems and needs (perhaps to the exclusion of other family members' needs), the whole family can eventually get worn down.

Since you, the family, are reading this chapter, it is perhaps best, if you have not done so, to go back and read the rest of the book up to this point before going on. If you do this, you will find yourself with a better understanding of your family member with pain and the general approach suggested here for coping with chronic pain. This understanding will enable you to better follow the rationale for changes which are recommended for *your* behaviour.

The most common (and very normal) family response is generally one of two—over-protectiveness or isolation and denial of the problem. Unfortunately, both of these natural

134

ways of handling the situation can, over time, serve to aggravate the family's and patient's problems further.

Over-protective Family Pattern

Lyn, a 28 year-old woman, had suffered since age twelve from back pain, apparently due to a malformation of her spine. Her parents had been very understanding with their only child. Lyn's mother gave up her job as a nurse to stay home and care for her daughter. Lyn and her mother engaged in many activities together but nothing strenuous. Sewing, games and music were the favourites. Lyn's mother also took charge of the pain medication, giving Lyn injections of analgesics when she needed them. As she was unable to do things with other children, Lyn had no social life outside the home.

By the time Lyn reached adulthood, the pattern was fully entrenched. Lyn's parents had turned their garage into a flat for her and she spent most of her time there. Mother and daughter argued constantly over medication—Lyn always wanting more and her mother trying to keep medication under reasonable control. Lyn's mother still spent hours entertaining her daughter, who, nevertheless, was often moody and irritable. When Lyn had a particularly bad night, which became a frequent occurrence, her mother would come out to the garage and sleep with her.

At 28, Lyn had never had a boyfriend and still had no girlfriends. When it was suggested to her that she should try becoming more socially active, she felt panicky, since she had no idea how to go about it.

Lyn's father, who had once participated in caring for her, driving her to and from music lessons or the doctor's office, became less sympathetic as Lyn grew older. Lyn's mother, however, continued with as much support and over-protection of her daughter as ever, and became angry when suggestions were made that Lyn should do more for herself. Again and again the mother mentioned how she had given up a nursing career to devote herself to her sick daughter.

The over-protective family pattern is one in which one or more family members assume the 'sick' person's family duties and responsibilities, so that the disabled family member doesn't have to 'overdo' it (that is, engage in activities which might cause pain). The chronic pain patient may, in effect, be 'policed' by other family members and scolded for doing too much, while at the same time he is told that he is privileged by this protection.

This family interaction has a way of forcing the chronic pain patient into greater and greater retirement, so that after a good deal of time has passed, he may, in fact, become more and more an invalid. But the process is a gradual and a subtle one. The assumption of the patient's family duties is usually gradual, with the patient slowly giving over more and more of his former role to the other family member(s). So slowly does this happen that no one is really aware of the changing family structure.

Often family members involved mutually reinforce this sort of over-protection. The patient is generally relieved to be excused from activities that he considers potentially painful (such as washing dishes, making beds, cleaning the cupboards, mowing the lawn, washing the windows or taking the kids to piano lessons). He even praises those who do the over-protecting: 'What would I do without you?' 'You're a good little helper.' 'You're so good to me.' 'Robert's a big help with the housework.' Friends of the family, relatives and neighbours also often give high praise to the over-protective family:'Isn't it great that Doreen's family understands?' 'You're very lucky that your family helps you out.'

On the other hand, there is also punishment inherent in adopting this family pattern. The sick family member feels guilty that he cannot fulfil his familial obligations. Moreover, the family members who take on the extra responsibilities will feel resentful from time to time, especially when the obligations interfere with some other preferred activity. These frictions inevitably lead to arguments, recriminations, and then more guilt. For a more complete explanation of this, the reader is referred back to the Take It Easy Trap and the Complaint-Resentment-Guilt Trap sections of Chapter 2.

In summary then, the main features of the over-protective

family pattern are prohibition of the pain patient from doing certain activities (which other family members then assume), an outward show of sympathy and understanding (with occasional, underlying feelings of anger or resentment), and guilt ('I'm not pulling my weight in the family.' 'What kind of person am I if I'm angry with a sick person?').

Isolation and Denial of the Problem

Carolyn, a 34 year-old farmer's wife had acquired back pain after a fall from a tractor. At the time of the fall, the marriage was only six months old. Ron, her husband, had been recently widowed with four teenage children. Carolyn, who had no children of her own, had been divorced several years earlier and had been working as a secretary in the city until she married Ron.

After her injury, the family was initially attentive, but as her back pain became chronic, the family increasingly began to show lack of concern, at least in Carolyn's view. Ron became more and more engrossed in his business. They stopped going out in the evenings. Ron had developed the habit of denying illness by losing himself in work years before, when his first wife had become chronically ill. Now he resumed the pattern. The children were involved in school and social activities and Carolyn felt they expected her to be their slave despite her pain problem. She complained that they made demands for meals at certain times so that they could get to this or that event with their friends, and they expected the right shirt or jumper to be clean and ironed when they wanted it. She felt unaccepted as their new mother. Coming from the city, Carolyn had enjoyed an active social life after her divorce, and now she found the isolation of the farm and the routine of household duties lonely and boring.

Although Carolyn tried repeatedly to express her problems, Ron refused to discuss them. He put her off with assurances that everything would work out if she just gave it time.

On three occasions recently she had been hospitalized with screaming episodes of pain. Ron became worried when this happened, stroking her hair soothingly all the way to the hospital in the ambulance. These episodes also brought more sympathy and concern from the children.

137

Carolyn was very aware that much of her problem had to do with her husband's lack of understanding and refusal to listen to and accept her problems of loneliness and feelings of being unappreciated. But whenever Carolyn tried to explain this to Ron, he only became angry at the doctors, insisting that there must be surgery which could help his wife.

In this family pattern, the patient's pain problem is generally ignored or denied—except when, on occasion, it gets so bad that it just can't be ignored. The family is then forced to pay attention to it. But, for most of the time, not only the pain is ignored, but all the other aspects of the patient's life— conversation, activities, interests, dreams and goals. In short, the patient, along with the pain, is ignored and denied. Avoidance becomes the primary way the family learns to deal with problems. For example, if the wife has chronic pain, the husband may become more and more engrossed in his work or business, spending progressively more time away from home. The children, following the example of the father, may become more involved in extra-curricular activities. Then the only time the patient can get attention is when she has a severe pain episode. If it is bad enough, it may be effective in keeping the husband and children home from work or play and getting them to show concern.

Patients with such family patterns often report that they usually don't bother to complain of pain since no one listens anyway. Unfortunately, this can lead to more dramatic gestures or cries for help—more frequent severe attacks or demonstrations of pain requiring hospitalization, frequent accidents or even, in very severe cases, overdoses of pain medication. Since normal complaining is ignored and since the patient's well behaviour, interests and activities are all ignored as well, the patient has no way to get the degree of attention that everyone needs. If it is only when he is very sick that concern is shown, the family is systematically training the patient that the only way to obtain attention, concern and love is by *being* very sick. In this case it is no wonder that a patient begins having more frequent, severe pain episodes. This may sound as if the patient is having pain attacks for the *purpose* of getting attention. This is definitely not the case. The pain is not being made up, willed, or exaggerated. The pain is *real* and the pain *is* worse during severe episodes. What is true, though, is that the pain is worse because the family environment has responded to the pain in such a way as to cause the severe pain episodes to be *learned*. The next section will help clarify this phenomenon.

Pain as a Learned Response

It is often difficult for people to understand how bodily responses or sensations can be learned. Most people think only outward behaviour is learned. In fact this is only part of the story, since not only behaviour, but also thoughts and even bodily responses can be learned. An analogy may help.*

If you see your favourite food when you are hungry (say a steak sizzling on a barbeque), you will salivate. That is, if your saliva were measured at that time, you would find that you were producing more saliva than you normally do. However, had we run this same test on you as a baby, before you had ever tasted grilled steak, no extra salivation would have occurred. The creation of extra saliva is a *learned,* physical, bodily response. Your *body* has learned to recognize steak as a tasty food, and it is this learning which now causes an automatic, physical reaction in you. Food which you do not like (such as the fried grasshoppers eaten in some parts of the world) would not cause you to salivate. It might even make you feel nauseous. The feeling of nausea is a *physical sensation,* but also a *learned* one. No one doubts the reality of that extra saliva or the nausea, and they are *learned* responses. Similarly, there

*This footnote is for more technically minded readers. It should be noted that the example supplied is one of learning by classical conditioning, while most pain behaviour, in fact, seems to be learned via operant conditioning. It is presented, however, simply as an example of a bodily response which is subject to learning, with the assumption that it is a more easily understood example than other operant analogies.

should be no doubt that, under certain circumstances, pain, too, can be learned, and it is just as real. Learned pain is, essentially, no different than pain due to an active injury. Only the origins differ. In fact, it is thought that pain which initially results from an injury can end up being learned, so that it persists long beyond the healing of the injury. The learned pain may be just as severe or even worse than the first onset of pain. And it is certainly just as real.

The Maladaptive Family Learning Patterns

The two family styles described above represent the extremes. More often families arrive at some mixture of over-protection and denial. You were probably able to recognise some aspect of your own family's style in these brief descriptions. The important thing to be noted, however, is that in both patterns the family environment ends up causing pain to be *learned*. In both cases or in mixtures of the two, pain behaviour is being reinforced and normal behaviour is being punished or ignored. In the over-protective family, pain behaviour (such as withdrawal from activity, resting, etc.) is reinforced by the family (by taking over the patient's tasks, giving sympathy, etc.), while non-pain or normal behaviour is punished or prohibited (the patient is kept from assuming normal responsibilities). In the isolation and denial family style, pain behaviour (severe pain attacks) are reinforced by the family's expression of concern and normal behaviour is ignored or at least fails to receive the usual rewards or appreciation which would maintain it. Some pain behaviour (minor complaints) is ignored but more severe pain *is* reinforced. Both of these family patterns ultimately promote the continuance of the Chronic Pain Trap since they promote the body's *learning* of the pain sensation as a more frequent and more intense experience.

Another of the subtle changes that families often learn as they adjust to chronic pain involves a rearrangement of roles within the family. If the wife and mother is the chronic pain patient, an older child or the husband may become the 'mother' to the family—the one who makes household decisions, disciplines the younger children or comforts them in their sorrows. If a working or professional woman becomes a chronic pain patient, the new dependence on the husband may throw both of them off balance. If the husband and father of a family is the chronic pain sufferer, the wife may take over some of his roles as 'bread-winner' and decision-maker, while older children take over his household responsibilities. He may adopt the role of 'house-husband'. Such role changes often become entrenched and may be difficult to reverse. Any family pattern is difficult to break since it involves habits that the *whole family* has adopted. This means that any change has to be brought about by changing the behaviour pattern of every member of the family.

How to Change Maladaptive Family Learning Patterns

Nancy, the 17 year-old daughter of Ann, whose case was described on pages 14-15 and followed up on page 46, had taken complete charge of the housework as well as the care of her younger sister as her mother had become slowly incapacitated. Initially, Nancy complained about her heavy chores, but as her social life and demands from her peers diminished as she became more and more busy after school, she slowly adjusted. Although Ann supervised and frequently criticised her work, she also praised her daughter, saying that she didn't know how she would get along without her. Nancy's father, who also gave compliments sparingly, praised Nancy for her housework. Her younger sister, on the other hand, rewarded her by irritating her constantly by such things as invading Nancy's room or borrowing precious possessions without permission.

When Ann began improving in the amount of activity she could do as described on pages 46-7, she was surprised to discover that when she tried to resume her role as housekeeper and mother, she was running into resistance from Nancy. Although Nancy still complained about housework, her role as mother of the family obviously paid off in some ways. Also, Nancy no longer had an active social life to return to, having given that up years before.

Ann solved the problem of shifting roles by allowing her daughter to take a part-time job after school so that she could begin saving money for university. By removing Nancy from the house at critical times, Ann was able to resume her former role and Nancy was provided with a new role. Nancy's parents were able to praise her for her part-time job and growing bank account; this praise replaced that which she had previously received in her role as substitute mother to the family.

The most important way in which a family can change is to change the focus from what the patient can*not* do to what he *can* do. This may require you, the family members, to do several things differently:

1. Stop taking responsibility for the chronic pain sufferer's activities. You should no longer forbid or discourage him from certain activities. He will know what he can and can't do and can decide for himself. If he does something you think he shouldn't do, it's better to keep quiet. If he suffers pain later, don't say: 'I told you so.' Don't even mention it. He is engaging in a retraining programme which will require effort and perhaps, from time to time, some discomfort. In the long run it will pay off.

2. Notice, praise or compliment him when he engages in *normal* activities. Normal activities may include many things: getting dressed by himself, making dinner, going out for an evening, sewing or building something, writing a letter, doing dishes, visiting a friend or going shopping. It is of critical importance that you give attention to the chronic pain sufferer's normal behaviour. This is not being patronizing. After all, it is an effort for him to do things normally and this effort should not go unnoticed. This is where most families fall down. They are so busy noticing and attending to the things the patient can't do that his successes go unnoticed. You have to turn the tables and begin noticing and praising achievements. If achievements are acknowledged they will be laboured for with even more effort. And anyway, you *do* appreciate the nice dinner which has been cooked for you, the jumper which was

knitted for you, a freshly mowed lawn, or having the company of your spouse at your boss's party, don't you? Why not say so? We sometimes act as if praise has to be artificial, unnatural or only for children. *We all need praise!* We all need to be told that certain things we do please others and are appreciated. It's how praise is given that makes it seem genuine or artificial. Praise, or noticing and thanking someone for doing something, can be very natural and genuine. Telling someone who has made an effort to look nice that they do look nice, handsome, beautiful, that you like their new hairstyle or new shirt, takes little effort. Saying that you enjoyed a meal can be done in a hundred ways (a hug and a kiss; 'That was the best meal I've had in ages'; or 'Gee, Mum, the potatoes were good'). All that is being asked of you is that you *notice* normal behaviour and appreciate the effort. You will find that if you are successful at doing this, the pain patient will begin noticing the efforts *you* are making, and you will be back on the road to reciprocity which was discussed in Chapter 2. Moreover, you will be helping to actually eliminate the symptoms of chronic pain. Normal behaviour and activity replaces 'sick' or 'pain' behaviour and lifestyle. One can't look well groomed and unkempt at the same time, can't be cooking dinner and in bed at the same time.

3. The third thing you can do is to help the patient avoid talking about his pain or problems. Your family member with chronic pain, if trying to follow the programme in this book, has been told not to discuss and not to think about his pain or problems. The rationale for this is that focusing on pain and problems makes them worse. If he can think pleasant, instead of dreary thoughts, think about something he is doing rather than how badly he feels, then he will feel better more of the time. To some extent, what one focuses one's thoughts and conversations upon controls how badly one feels. While he may continue to feel pain even if he doesn't talk or think about it, its effect on how badly he feels or suffers will be less with his focus diverted to more normal

conversation and activity. Have you ever noticed that if you have a pain of some sort—perhaps a headache or toothache—and you get absorbed in a particularly exciting movie or book, your mind escapes into that diversion and although you still feel the pain, you don't notice it as often or as intensely as you do when you're lying in bed trying to go to sleep with nothing else to think about. Well, the same principle holds true here.

Since thinking or talking about pain, treatment procedures (such as medication, the latest operation, what the physiotherapist did today) or other problem-related subjects, has usually become a fairly common occurrence with chronic pain sufferers, it may be a particularly hard habit to break. It is important that you do not bring up such topics, and if your partner does, gently remind him not to discuss it. Avoid asking how he feels. Ask instead about what he's been doing, what he thinks about such and such, what exercises he did today, or who he talked with.

The best way to initiate this new interaction pattern is by setting up an agreement between the two of you. You agree together to change your habits. This way your partner doesn't feel that you are imposing something on him. Discuss with him how you can best help him not to talk about pain and problems. Then stick to your joint agreement.

A very important word of warning: this suggestion should not be attempted unless you have made a genuine effort to put into effect the second suggestion listed on page 142. Families always seem to find it easy to stop discussing pain, but they often forget or feel foolish about noticing and praising normal, 'well' behaviour. But if you ignore discussion of pain and problems *without* attending to normal behaviour, you will end up with the family pattern and problems described under 'Isolation and Denial of the Problem' mentioned on page 137. The big difference is the *shift* of family attention, away from the problems and onto normal living. And remember that you should be patient in your efforts. Change will be gradual. It is important not to expect rapid change since you are working with very well-established behaviour patterns. They have taken a long time to learn; it will take some time to unlearn them.

4. Shifting the family focus away from pain and other problems often leaves family members wondering what they *are* going to talk about. You can't be praising 'well' behaviour *all* the time. But there are many other positive, happy aspects of life that you can make the focus of your conversation. Given the dominance of pain in your family's life, you just haven't been talking about such things recently. To help you get started again, some suggestions are made below.

a) Tell the chronic pain patient about *your* activities. Confide in him what's happening to you when you're out of his presence. This allows him to get interested in what you are doing and to eventually be able to ask questions. Often spouses or other family members don't bother to tell the pain patient about their activities or problems. Unfortunately this serves only to isolate him further.

b) Ask, and make sure you hear, what the pain patient has been doing. Often pain patients stop telling you about the events and activities in their lives for fear of boring you with all your more 'important' or 'interesting' things to think about. Show interest. Follow up with questions. Be sure to really listen.

c) Identify some areas of common interest that you can enjoy discussing together. You may find it helpful to fill out ten items each on the **Mutually Interesting Conversation Topics** worksheet (see page 146), comparing notes afterward. Topics that you both list will be good material for interesting, two-way conversation. If, however, you have trouble matching up topics, perhaps you need to generate some new common interests. You can do such things as reading together, taking a class together or joining the same club. Joint activities invariably lead to a growth in common interests.

Mutually Interesting Conversation Topics

List conversation topics that you think interest both of you. Fold the page over on the centre line and fill in your items independently. Then compare notes. Be sure to confirm with one another that topics listed really are of *mutual* interest. There's no point in boring each other. Continue working until you arrive at ten topics of mutual interest.

Patient's List	Partner's List

d) Make future plans together. Often pain patients and their families don't make plans since they feel that the future is so uncertain. But now that you have decided to give up further surgeries, hospitalizations and other time-consuming treatments, and you have embarked on the road to rehabilitation, it is time to start making plans again. Let your imagination go. Without things to look forward to, it is very difficult to be happy. Plans and dreams are often long term projects.

They may be such things as a long desired holiday to a place you've never been, buying some land, building your own house, buying camping equipment or a boat. Even allow yourself to share some dreams which may seem almost impossible to achieve. We all need a little fantasy. Modern life does not afford us much, but fantasy dreams are good for you too. You will be aware of the difference. Have some realistic plans and some fantasy dreams. Who knows? In time, even fantasy dreams may come true. The important thing is to determine some mutual plans to talk about. A great deal of enjoyment can be obtained from discussing these prospects.

5. If the pain patient in your family follows the advice on building activity gradually but systematically, as explained in Chapter 5, he will gradually be able to do more. As activity is increased in this structured way, it is important to *apply* the gains more generally by starting gradually to do more practical things. These practical things don't all have to be burdensome duties; practical activities might be fun, recreational pastimes as well. In fact, it is important that old activities which were once enjoyed are reinstated in your partner and family member's life. You may enjoy them as well! After all, many recreational activities in which the family can participate together, or which you and your partner can do together, have probably long gone by the wayside. Now that his standing and sitting activity is increasing, why not begin doing some of these things again?

Activities which have been neglected for months or years often end up being completely forgotten. It sometimes takes some hard thinking to remember all the things that you used to enjoy doing. Just to get you started, page 148 provides a list of activities that other chronic pain sufferers have resumed as part of their programmes. Go through the list together and make a mark by the ones which you think your family or you as a couple might enjoy together. When making up your own list draw especially from activities which you enjoyed in the past, or propose things that you used to talk about but that you never got around to doing. You might even want to add a couple of things which may seem quite foreign to you but which could possibly be fun.

Family Activity Programme (Part 1)

Below you will find suggestions for recreational activities for you as a family and you as a couple. Make a mark beside those which interest you, then add these and others to your own list.

Activities for the Whole Family

Going for a picnic

Camping

Attending a football, cricket or rugger game

Going to a film

Walking in the park

Shopping (for toys, sports equipment, family hobbies, etc.)

Eating at a restaurant or pizza parlour

Driving in the country

Swimming

Going to the zoo

Flying a kite

Planting a garden

Having breakfast out

Playing chasings, kicking a football or playing another game

Couple Activities

Reading a book together

Going to a film

Going to a concert or play

Playing golf, tennis or some other sport

Going away for a weekend

Shopping (or window shopping)

Taking a class together (e.g. cooking, a foreign language, painting, pottery, etc.)

Joining a club or group (e.g. football, church group, dance group, political group, etc.)

Going out to dinner

Family Activity Programme (Part 2)

Over the next four weeks, plan one activity per week from each list. Note date, activity, what planning must be done ahead and whose responsibility it will be to carry out the preliminary planning.

Week	Date	Activity for the Whole Family	Planning & Person Responsible
1.			
2.			
3.			
4.			

Week	Date	Couple Activity	Planning & Person Responsible
1.			
2.			
3.			
4.			

Once you have completed your lists, make specific plans

for how and when you will actually begin engaging in the activities that you have chosen. Make out a timetable for the next month. Try *at least one* activity from each list *every* week. In the **Family Activity Programme** worksheet (Part 2) on page 149 you will see that activities are planned for the next four weeks. In your own worksheet write down the date when you plan a given activity. On the right of that, note what preliminary planning, if any, has to be done to get things organized. For dinner at a restaurant, for example, reservations may have to ·be made; for a football game, tickets will have to be bought; for building something, materials will have to be purchased. Also make a note of who will be responsible for each of these preliminaries.

Once the plans are made, they should take precedence over *anything* else. And you should follow through regardless of how either of you is feeling. Pain, anger or anything else should not be used as an excuse to change or drop your plans. It is essential that neither of you lets the other one down by not following through on these activity plans. If you, the patient, are not feeling well, go along anyway. You will probably find that as you get involved in the activity, you will begin to feel better. And, you the family, don't forget to acknowledge your pleasure at the pain sufferer's participation in activities with you. Finally, during family activities, always try to keep the conversation on positive, happy things.

6. Help your partner gradually to resume his old role in the family. This may mean encouraging the children to go to him with their problems, or putting certain decision-making tasks back into his realm of responsibility. Role changes are often subtle things and need to be carefully analysed before it can be determined which duties or responsibilities have shifted over to other family members. Don't overlook the simple things, such as deciding on the grocery list, what to have for dinner, writing cheques, being the family budget-keeper, depositing money in the savings account, filling out the tax forms, filling the petrol tank, being the one who

disciplines the children, initiating sex or being the one who decides on this year's holiday spot.

The task of readjusting family role responsibilities must be tackled mutually, since everyone will have to agree on which duties are to be returned to the chronic pain family member and on what schedule. Since the responsibilities were relinquished gradually, the shift back should be made gradually. Probably the best way to start is to make up a mutually agreed upon list, ordering items in terms of difficulty and proposing target dates for resumption of responsibilities. Remember though, that a family member who has gained a role responsibility often finds it hard to turn it back over. So, be sensitive and be ready to do some mutual negotiation. You may have to make compromises or other accommodations.

Summary

Rehabilitation from the problems of chronic pain requires changes in the habits of everyone in the family. Several ideas for constructive change have been suggested here. Begin sharing more enjoyable activities. Focus more of your conversation on happy, positive things, such as each person's outside activities, mutual topics of interest or future plans and goals. This doesn't mean that you should *never* discuss problems or unpleasant issues (although you should avoid discussing the pain problem itself as much as possible), but the emphasis of most family conversation should be shifted away from problems. The pain patient should be encouraged, not discouraged from engaging in all sorts of activity. Normal functioning should be noticed and appreciated. And finally, an effort should be made to return old family role responsibilities to the patient.

These recommendations are not always easy to implement. Use the worksheets in this chapter to help you get going. Frequent review of your progress and occasional re-reading of this chapter may also be of assistance. However hard it is to get started, you will find that the programme becomes much easier once you are into it. And this is true, at least in part, because the practices outlined in this chapter lead to a much healthier family interaction and thus to a happier life for all concerned.

10. Preventing Pain

Much of this book is directed toward helping you to control your response to pain. And, in fact, doing this often leads to less pain. But there is another way that pain can be prevented and that is through muscle relaxation. As noted at various points in the previous chapters, muscle tension is a common cause of pain. It can also aggravate existing pain problems. Therefore, learning and practising relaxation techniques can be an effective preventive measure.

While we have good control over some muscles in our body, such as hand muscles, which can be tensed and relaxed at will, other muscles, such as those in the head, neck or back are not so directly in our control. The latter types of muscles can build up tension to such a point that they begin to hurt, often before we realize what is happening. When they are actually causing pain, it can be difficult to quickly remedy the situation. Assuming that the right muscles can be sorted out, relaxing them at this point is no guarantee that the pain will go away immediately. The muscles may now be sore and, even in a relaxed state, can still hurt from the long period of tension which preceded the pain. Obviously then, the best way that relaxation can help is for it to be used *before* the muscles become so tense that they begin causing pain. So, you first have to relax this area regularly.

If you suspect that some of your pain is caused by muscle tension, your doctor or physiotherapist should be able to confirm it for you. They can also help you to identify the precise muscles or muscle groups that are at the root of the problem. Muscles that are causing this sort of pain are usually more prominent than normal since they are being given exercise through frequent tensing; therefore, a simple examination can, in most cases, easily pinpoint the trouble spots.

The most common sites of muscle tension pain are the head, the shoulders and the neck. Tightness at any of these places can result in that familiar malady we call a headache. Pain may also be felt in the upper back or in more specific, localized areas. The following sections will give detailed instructions for exercises designed to relax head, shoulder and neck muscles, since these areas are the ones most people find troublesome. However, the same principles apply to procedures for relaxing muscles elsewhere in the body.

The exercises you are about to learn involve first tensing the muscle group, then relaxing it. The tensing is to help you identify the correct muscles and to help you to learn to discriminate more clearly between the feelings of tension and the feelings of relaxation. Eventually, once you become adept at relaxing, you will no longer need to do the tensing part of the exercise. You will be able to maintain a relaxed muscle state in areas that now cause problems.

These exercises only take a couple of minutes and can be done anywhere. The first few times, you may wish to do them in a relaxing, distraction-free environment so that you get the full benefit and learn the procedures well. After that, however, they should be practised *often,* throughout the course of your daily activities. They can be done while standing or sitting, working or at rest.

Forehead Tension

Two sets of muscles in the forehead and temple area (the
154

frontalis and temporalis muscles) cause some people headaches. If you think this may be your trouble area, try working on the following exercises:

1. Wrinkle your forehead into a frown. Notice the pull of the muscles across your forehead and the sides of your head. Hold this tense position for five seconds. Now relax to a normal position. Notice the muscles unwinding and relaxing. Allow them to relax for thirty to forty-five seconds. Focus on the nature of the relaxed feeling in that muscle group. Repeat if these muscles are not fully relaxed.

2. Raise your eyebrows high, which will stretch your forehead and other head muscles. Concentrate on the feeling of tension and hold the position for about five seconds. Now relax to a normal position. Feel the muscles relax across the forehead and side of the head. Repeat if full relaxation of this muscle group is not achieved.

If tensing or relaxing causes you more pain, it may actually be a good sign. It probably means that you have chosen the correct muscle group.

Jaw Tension

Strange as it may seem, a number of headaches, as well as forms of facial pain, seem to be caused by people unconsciously clenching their teeth and tightening their jaw muscles (called masseters). Often people are aware that they do this, but they don't realize that it may be the source of their pain. Try clenching your teeth and put your hand alongside your jaw. You should be able to feel the muscle moving. Now that you have identified where it is, try clenching your teeth while looking in the mirror. If your jaw muscle pops out and is quite noticeable, this could be your problem area. Monitor yourself during the day to see whether you are tensing your jaw muscles. If you decide this could be a problem area, try the following exercise:

Clench your teeth for five seconds, taking careful note of the

155

feeling of tension in that area. Now relax the muscle. Focus your concentration on the muscle as it relaxes. Allow it to continue the relaxation process for thirty to forty-five seconds. If, at the end of this period, you feel that the muscles are still taut, start over and do the exercise again.

Neck and Shoulder Tension

One of the more common culprits in the neck and shoulder region is the trapezius muscle, which runs across the shoulders, up the neck and across the back of the head to the top. If you have neck or shoulder pain on occasion or if your pain begins in the neck or the back of your head and radiates upward, you have reason to suspect this muscle. Sometimes stress on the trapezius and other muscles in the area may actually be triggering the tension. A pillow which is not correct for you or the wrong posture may cause a strain which results in muscle spasms. Tasks such as driving, typing or other jobs in which you are required to hold your hands in front of you for long periods of time can also strain this muscle. Sometimes simple adjustments, such as changing a pillow, posture or the height of a chair when typing can eliminate this strain and therefore the pain. But if such changes do not work for you, you may wish to learn exercises in this area so that frequent regular periods of relaxation are introduced to counteract the strain, keeping the tension within normal limits.

There are four types of exercises to relax the neck and shoulders. They should be especially helpful if you have tension headaches. However, if you wear a neck brace or have an active neck injury, such as a whiplash, be sure to check with your doctor before doing them.

1. To tense your neck area, bring your head forward until your chin almost touches your chest. Now prevent it from doing so by pretending that there is a force pushing it away from your chest. Struggle against this force. Doing this should make all of your neck muscles tense. Sustain this for about five seconds, then relax your neck and return it to a normal

position. It takes several seconds for muscles to fully relax. Notice the relaxation process. Allow it to go on for about 30–45 seconds, then take careful note of the feeling of the muscles in their relaxed state. If your muscles do not feel fully relaxed, repeat the tension and relaxation pattern once again.

2. Move your head backwards as far as it will comfortably go. Tense your neck as you do so. Hold the tension for about five seconds. Notice what the tense muscles feel like. Now relax the muscles and return the head to a normal position. Allow the relaxation to continue for about thirty to forty-five seconds. Notice how different the same muscles feel when they are relaxed. If these muscles do not feel fully relaxed, repeat the process once more.

3. Move your shoulders together behind your back as if you were trying to make them touch each other. Notice the muscle tension this causes. Hold this pose for about five seconds. Now relax your shoulders and notice the difference. Allow the muscles to continue the relaxing process for thirty to forty-five seconds. Focus your attention on the feeling in the muscles. If these muscles do not feel completely relaxed, you may wish to repeat the cycle.

4. Hunch up your shoulders until they almost touch your ears. Feel the tension in your shoulders and neck. Keep this hunched position for about five seconds. Now relax to a normal position and let relaxation flow into the muscles. Notice what this feeling is like. Let your neck and shoulders relax for about thirty to forty-five seconds. You may repeat the process if necessary.

You may find that doing these exercises when you are in pain actually increases the pain a bit. If this is the case, it probably means that you have the right area and you need to be practising these exercises often. Remember that the exercises are not designed to lessen pain once you have it. They are meant to prevent pain from starting by keeping muscle tension levels under control. (Some people do, however, find that doing the exercises does relieve built-up tension and pain. While this is not the ideal way to use relaxation exercises, you may wish to try it, to see whether it works for you.)

Practising Relaxation

To be effective, relaxation exercises must be practised. There are two ways to schedule your practice. You can identify times to practice, such as every half hour for thirty seconds. Some people purchase kitchen timers or key chains with alarms to remind themselves (these can be carried in a handbag or briefcase or put in a desk drawer). Or you can relate your practising to events, such as every time the phone rings, every time you are stopped at a red light or every time you pass through a door frame. Either technique will work. The main point is to do something to *remind* you to practise. Muscle tension is often a problem for people who are busy—so busy they forget to practise. And busy people are the ones who probably most need the practice.

Your practice should be aimed at learning to quickly and easily relax the selected muscles, using the appropriate exercise(s). As noted above, the idea of these repeated tension-relaxation cycles is to help you to learn thoroughly the sensation of relaxation in those special muscles. How long this learning process takes varies from person to person, but with practice, it eventually comes to everyone. When it does, the process will become easier since you can then skip the tensing part of the exercise and go directly to the relaxation phase. Reaching this point will streamline and simplify your relaxation exercises, making it easy to schedule your practice even more frequently. Eventually it should become habitual. The people who really profit from this procedure in terms of freedom from previously suffered muscle tension pain are those who report that their relaxing has become automatic and unconscious because they have made such a habit of practising.

You are attempting to retrain your muscles. For years you

have been unconsciously training your muscles to be tense. It will take some convincing to get the message across to these muscles that relaxation is the new way of life. The key is practice—the more the better—hundreds of times a day, if possible, let that muscle go, release the tension in it, even if for only five seconds. The reward will be well worth it—the prevention of pain from muscle tension.

Biofeedback

If you find the relaxation procedure in this chapter unhelpful but you still think your problem is one of muscle tension, EMG biofeedback may be helpful. (EMG stands for 'electromyogram' which means the recording of electrical impulses coming from muscle activity.) EMG biofeedback is a procedure which many psychologists now use to treat problems such as tension headaches or neck pain. It involves several sessions of placing small electrodes on the troublesome muscles. These electrodes pick up the electrical potential in your muscles and transmit it to a biofeedback machine which sits in front of you, telling the exact level of tension or relaxation of that muscle. From this instant feedback from your body, you learn to discriminate between muscular tension and muscular relaxation. As you become better able to discriminate, you can begin practising the relaxed state. Moreover, as you practise, the biofeedback machine gives you constant and immediate feedback on how successful you are. Thus, you can adjust your efforts until you come upon techniques that work best for you.

Another type of biofeedback, called 'thermal biofeedback', also may be helpful in pain prevention for people who suffer migraine or 'cluster' headaches. These types of headaches are not muscle-tension based, but rather are thought to be related to the constriction and dilation of the blood vessels. The treatment involves using the biofeedback equipment to give you instant information on your skin temperature, which is related to blood-flow. Through this feedback, it is thought patients can learn to exercise some control over their vascular system and thus prevent the onset of conditions which create the headaches.

Biofeedback treatment is now available in many cities. If you call your local Pain Clinic (see Appendix), you should be able to get information on local practitioners who offer it.

Summary

In this chapter, it has been suggested that muscle tension is a condition which can result in episodes of pain. To prevent its occurrence, it is necessary first to identify the specific muscles or muscle groups which are the source of the problem. You may be able to make this judgement yourself, or your doctor or physiotherapist can assist you. Once the sites are determined, a schedule of relaxation exercises should be applied on a regular basis. If practised frequently enough, the exercises should lead to a generally more relaxed condition in the troublesome muscles—and pain from muscle tension will thus be avoided.

Forms of biofeedback treatment, available from psychologists, provide an alternative means to control muscle tension pain, as well as migraine and 'cluster' headaches. Biofeedback, however, involves a clinical rather than a self-help programme of treatment.

The forms of muscle relaxation listed here are directed at alleviating tension in specific, localized areas. There are, however, muscle relaxation programmes designed to help you with general relaxation. The interested reader is referred to the 'Further Reading' section on pages 189-202.

11. Recognizing and Solving Other Problems Which May Aggravate Pain

At age 62, Edna had suffered severe chronic back pain for five years, ever since the car accident that had left her paraplegic and had killed her retarded son. Edna's husband, who had been driving at the time of the accident, had escaped without serious injury. Edna had made a good adjustment to life in a wheelchair, learning to cook and take care of many other household chores independently, but she complained constantly of pain. The whole range of pain-killing drugs was tried, but even in strong doses they failed to give any relief. Edna reported that she had begun thinking about her pain nearly all the time. She complained bitterly to her husband and neighbours and cried easily and frequently. Her husband didn't know what to do and felt powerless.

Edna and her husband were taught strategies for focusing away from the pain and replacing negative thoughts and conversations with more positive, adaptive ones. With further exploration it became clear that Edna was suffering from problems other than pain—depression and anger. Throughout the five years, she had been depressed over her paralysis and her son's death and she held a grudge against her husband, whom she blamed for the accident. But she had avoided expressing these feelings for fear of angering her husband, upon whom she now felt more dependent than ever. Edna's pain complaints had been her only outlet for these cooped-up problems. The result had been to make her experience of pain all that much worse. And now, since the pain was all wrapped up with the depression and anger, it could not be dealt with alone.

People with chronic pain are not immune to other problems. Whatever other problems a person has in his life may have originated before or after the onset of chronic pain. It is not of great importance to know in what order problems arose, however, it is worth noting exactly what connections may have developed between such existing problems over the years. Clearly, no problem exists in a vacuum; problems often interact with one another, and generally, they can serve to aggravate or maintain each other. In some cases, one problem may work to help a person escape or avoid having to confront one or more other problems. This becomes a particularly difficult situation to resolve since the first problem serves a useful function in allowing the other to be avoided. This pattern is, in fact, quite common with pain. That is, pain can often provide a reason for avoiding other problems or uncomfortable situations. This is not to say that pain is *created* for the purpose of getting the patient out of something. Rather, it is simply that when pain and other problems exist side-by-side, the pain may eventually come to serve such a function.

There are, of course, many ways to avoid confronting problems (e.g. quitting a job, divorce or running away), but pain is one which is fairly socially acceptable. Being sick is viewed with sympathy in our culture, and certain allowances are made for the chronically ill person. In other words, the chronic pain patient can avoid facing up to other problems with little social pressure to do so. Very often patients are, themselves, unaware that their pain has come to function in this way. Even when the fear or anxiety created by the other problem(s) is very great, patients can overlook their existence. When questioned about what other problems they have, many pain patients report that they are not aware of any at all or at least none that they would label as serious. Often when the patient explores his life situation in more depth, he recognizes the existence of other such problems and begins to see them separately from his pain. In this circumstance, the pain has provided such an effective buffer against other problems that the patient doesn't even recognize that he has any problems other than the pain. Again, it should be stressed that this situation does not suggest that the pain exists for this purpose. It is merely that real pain has come to serve the function of helping the patient to avoid things that he is anxious about or which he finds unpleasant. There are, however, some very unfortunate consequences of pain coming to serve such a function. When pain repeatedly leads to avoidance of other problems, it can actually increase the severity of pain through learning. Moreover, any effort to reduce pain is going to result in having to face up to problems that may not have been confronted for a long time. So, it will be fighting an uphill battle. Indeed, the self-help programme outlined in this book may be difficult or impossible to follow since there could be something working against success—fear of facing some other problem(s). Therefore, it is all the more important for the chronic pain patient to do some serious thinking about what other problems he may have and what might be done about them, so that these don't end up maintaining or aggravating pain.

Problems which are more easily avoided than faced are many. Some of the most common are: sexual problems, marital or relationship problems, difficulty in relating to people, not being able to stand up for one's rights, failure to meet one's own or others' expectations, an intolerable job situation with little or no opportunity to change jobs, and alcohol problems. In addition, the stress of muscle tension and litigation often associated with chronic pain due to injury can also aggravate pain. These will be discussed below, one by one.

Sexual Problems

Ned, aged 41, had slowly and mysteriously (to him) become impotent over the previous few years. His wife, Marie, had suffered low back pain for a similar period. The couple avoided

163

sexual intercourse 'because of Marie's back'. When this was discussed with Marie in Ned's absence, she expressed relief that her back problem had kept Ned from having to face a loss of manliness due to what he viewed as sexual failure. By himself, Ned expressed fears that if she got better, Marie might place demands on him which he could not fulfil.

Fortunately, Ned and Marie accepted the suggestion of sexual counselling for their sexual problem after their doctor assured them that sexual intercourse could not further injure Marie's back. After several weeks of following the suggestions of the therapist, they happily reported that their sexual problem was solved. Although Marie still suffered from pain, she noted an improvement in her mood and an increase in self-confidence.

Ned and Marie were then ready to embark on the treatment procedures outlined in this book, having successfully solved one of the problems which may have aggravated the pain problem.

Many chronic pain patients and their spouses have sexual problems. In some cases these existed before pain became a problem; in others they began after the onset of pain. In either case, pain can become an excuse for not engaging in sexual activity, thereby helping the couple avoid confronting the sexual problem or the possibility of what is perceived as sexual failure.

It is not always the chronic pain patient who manifests the sexual problem; it is often the spouse. Of course, sexual problems are always problems for both partners. The most common sexual problems for men are impotence and premature ejaculation. For women, they are failure to achieve orgasm, vaginismus (difficulty accepting penetration due to muscle tension in the vagina) and dyspareunia (vaginal pain from intercourse). If couples live with such sexual problems for months or years, intercourse often becomes a time of tension and performance-anxiety, rather than pleasure. When this is the case, it may be easier to avoid sexual activity than to confront what you both may perceive as sexual failure on the part of one or both of you. Chronic pain can become a reason to avoid intercourse. Both partners state and believe that it is the pain which is causing them to avoid sexual activity. The fear of sexual failure or frustration is not openly acknowledged as contributing to sexual avoidance. Low back pain can become, for many couples, a permanent reason not to have intercourse—for fear of further injuring the patient's back or causing pain. Specific pain attacks, such as headaches, may become reasons why one partner just doesn't feel up to it. (The old joke: 'Not tonight, dear, I have a headache', may not be so funny.) This is a most unfortunate state of affairs for several reasons. Not only is the sexual problem helping to maintain the pain, but it is cutting off the patient and spouse from another pleasurable activity that they could enjoy together. Besides being enjoyable in and of itself, sexual intercourse can be an excellent mood elevator and can provide tension-release.

This situation is particularly sad since most sexual problems are *easily* solved these days. Since the work of Masters and Johnson (and now many others) there are many excellent behavioural treatment programmes for the sexual problems listed above. For example, the self-help book *Becoming Orgasmic: A Sexual Growth Programme for Women* by Julia Heiman, Leslie Lopiccolo and Joseph Lopiccolo tackles problems women have with achieving orgasm. Help can also readily be obtained for this and other sexual problems by contacting your local Pain Clinic (see Appendix) or your GP, or your nearest Marriage Guidance Council (see the telephone directory). Often only a few sessions of therapy can solve problems that you have lived with for years. Therapy usually involves the therapist suggesting a few exercises or specific instructions for things for you to engage in alone or with your partner in the privacy of your home. Many people are now availing themselves of this counselling and most find it helpful. If you prefer the self-help approach, the 'Further Reading' section (see page 193) suggests titles dealing specifically with sexual problems.

Pain should not become a reason for avoiding sexual intercourse. With some experimentation, most couples are able to work out satisfactory positions in which intercourse will not cause pain. If you are worried about causing your partner or yourself injury, check with your doctor. In most cases he will assure you that injury is almost impossible.

There is really no reason that you should not be enjoying a satisfactory sexual relationship. If sex does seem to present problems, seek help together and work on solving them. You will very likely be surprised at how easy the process is. If you have been avoiding sex simply for fear of pain or injury, experiment until you find ways in which you can both be satisfied without causing further pain. Perhaps you have been restricting your sexual habits too much. The *Joy of Sex* by Alex Comfort can be a helpful book to provide you with suggestions for alternate ways of giving and receiving pleasure. If you simply 'do not feel like it', give second thoughts to allowing yourself to participate anyway. As you will recall from the discussion in Chapter 8 concerning what you focus your attention upon, once you become interested and involved in an activity, your perception of pain will be lessened. What better distraction could there be than satisfying sex?

You should also be aware that sexual intercourse is one of those things that is better for both partners if practised often. When they do *not* engage in sexual activity frequently enough, men may lose control and women may find themselves less easily aroused. Thus, just by increasing your frequency, you can help resolve sexual problems and enjoy the activity more.

Finally, research has shown that in some non-orgasmic or seldom-orgasmic women, back pain can be caused by repeatedly being aroused without orgasmic release.

More generally, avoidance of sex causes any pain sufferer unnecessary sacrifice. It deprives you of that natural tranquillizer and anti-depressant that you may once have had more frequently.

Marital or Relationship Problems

Betty, a 70 year-old woman, had suffered rectal pain for the past seven years. Although she had been hospitalized twenty times, no treatment procedure (including surgery) had been successful for more than a couple of weeks. Due to pain, she was unable to walk more than a few steps at a time and could not sit at all, so that her activities were severely restricted.

Betty had been married to Clyde for 30 years—and they fought constantly. Everything each of them did irritated the other. They tried to control each other's every move. Since the pain greatly limited what Betty could do, Clyde had taken over caring for her and the household. And while both of them voiced literally hundreds of complaints about this arrangement, other evidence suggested that perhaps the arrangement was what they really wanted. She was outraged, for example, when he took a day off to go fishing. He criticised every attempt she made to become less dependent, even condemning simple tasks such as making jelly or making her bed.

At the same time, both parties were very hurt by their constant verbal attacks on each other. Each defended her or himself with even more bitter recriminations.

Openly and repeatedly, Betty voiced the opinion that her rectal pain was caused by Clyde. 'He's the *real* pain in the . . ,' she would say vehemently. She maintained that her frequent hospitalizations were partially to obtain a break away from him; she usually asked that Clyde's visiting hours be restricted even more than hospital rules allowed.

Betty and Clyde had a marital problem that aggravated the pain problem.

Intimate human relationships are always very complex. Once we know or live with a person for a long time, we develop fairly standard patterns of interaction. We learn what to expect from them so that, often, we can even predict their behaviour. Sometimes the established interaction pattern gives us what we need from the relationship—love, affection, companionship or attention. Other times it does not. In this case, we call it 'maladaptive'. Couples often have some of each—some adaptive and some maladaptive interaction patterns. The problem is to sort out the maladaptive patterns and to understand how they interact with the pain problem.

There are a number of possibilities. Pain may be used as a desperate attempt to hang onto the other person and keep him or her from leaving the relationship. ('If I didn't have you, I don't know what I'd do. I think I'd commit suicide.') Often one member of a couple, fearful that the other is unhappy or unsatisfied in the relationship, intensifies pain behaviour to hold on to the partner through guilt and sympathy. Pain behaviour may also serve to provide a reason that the pain patient is not meeting the other's needs. This can be a short-term solution to a marital problem, but it usually fails as a long-term solution. In fact, it may eventually help to *cause* the break-up of the relationship. Ultimately, most people will opt out of a relationship when there is a continuing lack of reciprocity. Of course, this is only one way in which pain can become a part of a relationship problem.

The best long-term solutions always involve facing up to whatever problems exist in your relationship, recognizing which of your behaviours need to be changed, and then active-ly working on it. If you wish to do this on a self-help basis, there are books which can be of help. See the section on marital problems at the back of the book under 'Further Reading'. Marital or relationship counselling can also be sought from the Marriage Guidance Council (see the telephone directory for your local branch), or from psychologists (your nearest Pain Clinic should be able to refer you appropriately). Some people are afraid of marital counselling. They fear that they will be blamed, or that the counsellor may side with the other partner. In fact, however, counsellors typically assume that problems are not the fault of either of you, but are, rather, interaction problems which can be solved by improved communication. Counselling can offer more direct communication skills, which will lead to more open expression of the needs of both partners, as well as the meeting of those needs. The same principles apply to counselling in relationship problems other than those of couples—for example, parent-child difficulties.

General Difficulty in Relating to Others

If a person has difficulty in relating to others, pain may become a reason for avoiding people. Some people have never been taught or had the opportunity to learn what psychologists call *social skills*—the ability to relate easily to others. Others have problems with *assertiveness*. There are two assertiveness problems—being too unassertive (so that others take advantage of you) or being too aggressive and pushy. In either case, you are likely to feel uncomfortable around others. You may feel that you can't form close relationships or that you can't talk to others. You may feel that people don't like you for yourself. You may feel uncomfortable with people of the opposite sex—unsure of what they want from you or how to approach them. All such problems can and do aggravate pain when pain becomes the excuse for avoiding the anxiety and discomfort associated with relating to other people. If you have pain, you are not expected to go out much or mix with others. You have a good excuse to stay home, an acceptable excuse. No one has to find out that you are uncomfortable with others and you don't have to be painfully reminded yourself. You avoid the problem. Since pain helps you do this, it becomes reinforced and increases its potential for being learned, as well as the probability that it will continue to be chronic.

These problems are also easily solved, and it is a shame not to work at resolving them since human relationships provide most people with their biggest source of joy and pleasure in life. Why cut yourself off just because you lack a few simple skills which can be easily learned?

Many social skill problems pivot around your either not feeling that you know the right thing to say at the right time or around your saying the wrong thing at the wrong time. Learning how to correctly evaluate a situation and what responses to make can be a matter of simply learning skills, followed by rehearsal and real life practice. Again, several books are available if you wish to tackle this problem on a self-help basis. They are listed in 'Further Reading—Assertive Problems'.

You can also work on these problems in therapy. Call a local Pain Clinic (see Appendix) for advice about therapists.

One general note on learning better social skills is that practice is important. The more you avoid interacting with others, the more awkward you will feel when you do have to do it. Practice will desensitize you and help you see that you *can* give and receive from others.

Failure to Live Up to Expectations

Susan, a 26-year-old medical secretary, had injured her back while skiing seven years ago. She had since undergone four operations, physiotherapy and traction, but nothing had worked to relieve the pain that had begun after the injury. Susan was the daughter of a wealthy Jewish family whose much-expressed goal for her was that she marry the 'right' boy and have children. Just before her skiing accident, however, these hopes seemed to be running into trouble. Susan had become pregnant, had an abortion, and shortly thereafter, she had dropped out of university. This series of events had greatly upset both Susan and her parents. Her parents felt that she had let them down and she felt so too. After her injury, however, her parents became very protective and began babying her, doing everything for her. Susan felt safe back in her parents' care. Due to her inactivity, she began putting on weight. This, her back pain and her frequent hospitalizations reduced her formerly active social life to nothing. She eventually took a job as a medical secretary, but her pain interfered with her work, causing her to be absent frequently.

As the years went by, Susan's parents gradually became resentful of her invalid role and began encouraging her to be active, to see friends and to go out. Susan however, was afraid of the dangers of independence and had by now become socially anxious, especially regarding men. At the same time, as she sat at home nightly with her hospital-style bed and hydroculator, watching TV, she continued to profess her desire to find the 'right' man and get married, just as her family had always wanted. In Susan's case, her failure to live up to her own and her parents' expectations was aggravating the pain.

The feeling that you are not living up to your own or someone else's expectations can also contribute toward maintaining your pain. In this case, pain becomes an acceptable reason for not meeting those expectations.

One of the most frequent instances in which expectations create problems seems to be when parents are involved. Parents sometimes place very powerful demands on children — these expectations may be unrealistically high, or even if easily achievable, they may not be what the child wants for himself. Nevertheless, we all want to please our parents, even long after we've grown to adulthood. Praise or criticism from them can still motivate us in many ways. Indeed, we often find that our parents' expectations, along with their praise and criticism have become internalized within us in a very real sense. Failure to achieve what we believe we should be able to do, according to these set expectations, can be a truly devastating experience for our self-concept. A pain problem, however, can provide a convenient reason, to oneself and to others, why one is unable to achieve the expected successes and glories.

Usually one does not live up to one's own or others' expectations for one of three reasons:

1. one does not possess the necessary skills,
2. one does not have the necessary motivation (parents' expectations or parent-instilled expectations and one's own desires may be in conflict), or
3. one has unrealistic expectations for oneself.

More often than not, reasons 2 or 3 are the culprits. If you analyse yourself and find either or both of these at fault, the obvious solution to your problem is to change your expectations to more realistic, reasonable ones. Of course, at the same time, you must reject the old ones, which were making you feel like a failure. It can, however, be a difficult process to reject unrealistic, perfectionist notions and to recognize oneself as only human. But it can be done. If you wish to tackle it on a self-help basis, *A New Guide to Rational Living* by Albert Ellis and Robert Harper can provide you with a beginning. (Other suggestions for further study are provided in 'Further Reading—Assertive Problems'.) Or you may find it easier to work on changing your self-expectancies and self-evaluations with the help of a psychologist. (Contact a local Pain Clinic for advice on how to find a psychologist.) You *can* change your negative self-evaluations and unrealistic expectancies. In the process you may learn how to be more self-sufficient in self-praise and self-criticism, and how to become less sensitive to the expectations and evaluations of others. If you do this, it will no longer be necessary for your pain to function as a means of avoiding situations in which you fear failure. With proper expectations, you won't have to worry about failure.

An Unhappy Job Situation

Sometimes people get trapped in jobs that they really hate. There are any number of reasons for hating a job; it may be too high-pressure, too boring, or it may bring you into contact with people you dislike. All too often, people feel that they are unable to do anything about an unhappy job situation. The family may depend on the earnings. It may seem impossible to take the necessary time off to retrain for another position. A worker may feel unable to move to a new job or he may feel he is too old to be hired anywhere else. However, chronic pain can become a reason to avoid work. In time, most chronic pain patients find themselves quitting their jobs. Retiring from work aggravates the problem in several ways:

1. it tends to reinforce the pain and contribute to pain becoming learned and therefore chronic;
2. it throws you into the Take It Easy Trap described in Chapter 2;
3. it can result in your receiving worker's compensation (if you were injured at work) and that can, in itself, cause a whole host of problems which will be discussed below;
4. financial problems may become worse than ever, and that can cause tension which further aggravates pain; and
5. your opinion of yourself is likely to suffer since you will not be living up to your ideas concerning the value and importance of work.

If you have chronic pain, if you are no longer working and if you hated or disliked your job, it is very possible that your problems interact in this way. You may not be aware of these interactions. Uncomfortable facts are easier to deny. However, whether you realize it or not, the overall pattern is probably reinforcing your pain and making it worse in the long run.

If the three 'ifs' above pertain to you, you have three choices:

1. return to the hated job, in which case you are likely to continue to become worse (so, in the end, you'll be forced to retire anyway),
2. get caught in the Chronic Pain Trap permanently, or
3. give a chance to a new career or less difficult job.

At the moment, you may believe that the third option is impossible. But is it really? Or are the barriers artificial?

If you don't like your job, the first thing to do is to admit to yourself and your family that you do hate it. There's no crime in that. Lots of people hate their jobs and it really is silly to stay for the rest of your life in a job that you hate. Work, after all, takes the most important part of most days, so why stick with an intolerable job situation? Hating one job doesn't mean that you will hate all jobs. In fact, this may be an excellent time to think of trying something new. Starting again may seem hard, but when compared to the difficulties of the Chronic Pain Trap, is it really? You may worry that it would put too much financial stress on your family, but compared to the strain, tension and upset of the Chronic Pain Trap, would it really? Chronic pain patients often find that as the years of retirement grind on, they are unable to enjoy life and become bored. Spouse and children often begin to question or openly dislike the fact that the patient doesn't work. The patient himself develops a bad opinion of himself, feeling that he has accomplished nothing, contributes nothing and is good for nothing. People begin to wonder whether the chronic pain has been fabricated in order to get compensation payments, and there are the continuing reviews and battles concerning whether or not compensation should be continued. Is it all really worth it?

There are alternatives, but they tend to be very individualized, so you will have to spend some time investigating what is right for you. A good way to begin is to remember what you've always thought you would enjoy doing. Analyse your personal strengths (e.g. good with people, good at figures, good with my hands, independent, imaginative, etc.) and compare your strengths with those required for the potential job. This is a good activity to share with your partner or another family member. Make a list of three potential alternative jobs that you could do if you had the right training. Do your homework and find out the minimum requirements for each job. Homework, in this case, may be going around and discussing jobs with personnel departments, ringing training institutions such as universities, technical schools or advanced colleges, talking with relatives or friends already doing the job, or working with a vocational counsellor. As a chronic pain sufferer, you may qualify as disabled and that could mean you are eligible for certain benefits. You should consult your doctor and Citizen's Advice Bureau, as well as the local Job Centre.

Remember not to make the same mistakes all over again; you are looking for a job that you like, or at the least, one you can tolerate. Don't repeat the mistake and end up with another boring or high-pressure job.

Starting a new career or changing jobs may involve doing several things which are difficult. It may mean changing your self-image as well as your family's image of you. If you've always thought of yourself as a teacher, naval officer, accountant or salesperson, the shift can be hard. You may be starting at a lower salary or having less prestige than you were accustomed to. You may even be starting your new job on just a part-time basis. Full-time or part-time, some adjustment in your compensation payment may have to be made. This does not mean, however, that your compensation will necessarily be cut completely. Often you and your insurance company can work out a partial compensation payment from your company to supplement a lower wage, if you have taken a cut in pay.

174

You may think that if you are a housewife and mother, this does not apply to you. But housewives and mothers can be just as unhappy with their work as anybody else, particularly if they have been doing the same thing for a very long time. Being a housewife and mother can be very gratifying, but it is only gratifying if you are cut out for it and if enough rewards and appreciation are forthcoming from the family. Just as every man is not cut out for the same job, so every woman may not enjoy continual housework and motherhood. Moreover, as with any job, the working conditions may change over the years and a once-rewarding job may become less enjoyable. Often as the children get older and eventually move out of the home, the housewife's job begins to seem empty or meaningless. But while the old job has lost its lustre, alternatives seem to be non-existent. Many women feel that they don't know how to do anything else or that they are too old to be employed. This is just not true. Perhaps it is more difficult if you are older, but it is *never too late to start something new*. And if you look hard enough, you *will* find something you can do. You may actually have an advantage in choosing another career later in life. You probably know yourself better and will be better able to predict the sorts of things you will like.

Once you make the choice of a new job, you may find that you need to have some special training. But this can be very enjoyable. Many people feel that they are too old to go back to school; they worry that they won't be able to handle it. In fact, this is almost always untrue; older students are often the best. They are more mature, more motivated, study harder and usually have more stable lifestyles than their younger competitors. If you choose to train in an area that can maintain your interest and if you allow yourself time to adjust to your new routine, your chances of success will be very good.

Remember, though, that this change of role can sometimes be difficult for husbands and families to adjust to. Husbands may have unrealistic fears about losing the attention they are used to or fears that they may lose their wives altogether to another man. Children sometimes worry that their mothers are going to withdraw the maternal love and support that they need. Usually, however, these fears vanish after a few months' exposure to the new situation. There may be a period of adjustment, resentment, spoken or unspoken dissent, but in the end, when the feared consequences do not materialize, attitude changes will come about. Moreover, if they take stock of the alternative—continuing in the Chronic Pain Trap—especially if they have read this book—your family members are likely to support your new direction. In fact, most people find their family relationship improves when the wife and mother is happier with her work.

The important point in all of this is that if you dislike your job—whether it is a paying job or housework—it is never too late to try out a new career. In the long run, it is much better for your health than remaining in a hated job, where the tension will aggravate your pain. It is also vastly better than premature retirement—with all of the accompanying dangers of the Take It Easy Trap, as described in Chapter 2. This may be a unique opportunity to rethink and re-begin an important part of your life. It may cost you something in income and prestige, but how unimportant these are compared to better health and happiness.

Alcohol Problems

Margaret, a 49 year-old housewife and former factory worker, suffered upper back and shoulder pain after a car accident. She and her husband had been fairly heavy social drinkers before the accident. When surgery, physiotherapy and medication all proved futile, Margaret began drinking vodka and gin to ease the pain during the day while her husband was at work. When he came home, she would continue drinking with him throughout the evening. Her husband was worried about the amount she was drinking since she was often inebriated when he came home. He cut back on his own drinking in an attempt to help her control hers. But Margaret told him that he didn't understand since he didn't suffer chronic pain. If she reduced her alcohol consumption, she argued, the pain would worsen. And she denied that she drank as much as he claimed anyway. For Margaret, pain and a drinking problem were helping to maintain each other.

Sometimes trouble with alcohol can be the 'other problem' which one manages to avoid facing. It can be very difficult to confront the fact that one's drinking is out of control. The very notion of being considered an 'alcoholic' may seem too painful to deal with. Even if you can admit to yourself that alcohol has become a problem, the thought of taking the usually accepted cure—to stop drinking— may seem even more painful and therefore something to be avoided. Chronic pain can provide what appears to be a good reason for not facing up to alcohol problems, especially if one uses alcohol as an analgesic. Patients often feel that if alcohol is used to kill or dull the pain, it can be considered acceptable to themselves and to their family. Additionally, the lifestyle of someone with chronic pain—not working, being inactive and unable to go out to social engagements—easily covers for the consequences of a drinking problem. Chronic pain is, after all, a much more acceptable reason for withdrawing from life than is 'alcoholism'. Again, it should be stressed that pain is not created or invented to serve this function, but rather pain may come to provide this service. Unfortunately, this useful function can only reinforce the pain, increasing its learning component and making it more likely that it will be unresponsive to treatment. Thus, chronic pain and problem drinking interact to make your situation worse and worse.

If this sounds familiar or if you use alcohol as an analgesic, you should realize that it is important for you to tackle your other problem—problem drinking—before or at the same time as you work on your pain problem. There are many ways to work on alcohol problems. If you want to try to do something on a self-help basis, you can read *How to Control Your Drinking* by William R. Miller and Ricardo Munoz, which is aimed at teaching you techniques for moderate instead of destructive drinking. There are many other treatment programmes for alcohol problems. Inquire by telephoning your GP, the nearest

Pain Clinic (see Appendix) or your local social services department. Alcoholics Anonymous (AA), also available in most communities and listed in your telephone book, still has one of the best success rates. AA's approach is total abstinence, using group techniques so that people with similar problems help each other.

No matter how you go about tackling an alcohol problem, it is necessary from the very beginning to separate your drinking from your pain problems. Stop using alcohol as an analgesic. Do not take it when you have a pain attack. Re-read Chapter 7, 'Controlling the Pain Killers' and Chapter 8, 'What to Do and What Not to Do When You Are in Pain'.

A word of warning: alcohol does not mix well with many other drugs and may be harmful or even lethal if taken along with medication. It is not unheard of for patients to accidentally kill themselves by not realizing which medications do not mix with drink or by deceiving themselves or their doctors about how much alcohol or how many other things they take. In this case, avoiding problems can be deadly.

Alcohol, of course, is not the only drug which can interact with pain in this way. The section on the Medication Trap in Chapter 2 and all of Chapter 7 have already discussed how continued use of prescribed drugs can not only reinforce pain, but become a problem in and of itself. Illegal 'street drugs' can also be involved in maladaptive interaction with chronic pain which can serve to continue both problems. However, regardless of the type of drug involved, the solutions recommended above and in Chapters 7 and 8 work equally well.

Litigation

Sometimes patients are injured in accidents at work, in a car or in some other circumstance deemed to be someone else's fault. In this case, the patient may be able to sue the other party. And, in fact, large numbers of people who suffer chronic pain at some point find themselves involved in a lawsuit or litigation.

However, the trouble with lawsuits is that they usually take a long time to settle—often years—and the patient is placed in the position of having to continue to *prove* how disabled he or she is during all that time. Subtle and not-so-subtle pressure is continually placed on the patient to remain sick and *in* chronic pain. The battle against the company or person, the constant examinations, re-examinations and certifications by various doctors and specialists all exert pressure to prove how disabled the patient is. The patient may be advised against appearing too well by his family or lawyer. He may be advised not to go to work, and not to appear to enjoy himself too much in his retirement. Obviously, all this works against rehabilitation. And whether or not the patient has any awareness of it, the pattern *reinforces* pain.

There are two other factors regarding litigation that can create problems. One is the tension involved. Being involved in legal action can be very tension-producing. The person who is suing wants to win; the person or company being sued doesn't want to lose. Contention and animosity arise; this leads to tension and tension, in turn, aggravates pain. The other factor concerns the sizable amounts of money over which suits are fought. The prospect of gaining a large award may be reinforcing in itself, not only to the patient, but also to his lawyer and family. Such reinforcement can serve to contribute to the learning component of pain.

The other side of the litigation problem is the suspicion that instantly crops up. Just being involved in a suit is enough to suggest to many people that you have reasons for wanting the pain to continue. This places you in the unenviable position of having others, whether they are involved in the litigation or not, believing that you are imagining or exaggerating the pain. Many doctors, for example, are automatically more suspicious of their patients' motives if the patients are involved in litigation.

Given all this, you must ask yourself whether it is worth it. Since being involved in the litigation process acts against your returning to a more normal lifestyle and works in favour of your continuing in the Chronic Pain Trap, is litigation really worth the trouble? Is anything, even money, worth losing your health and happiness? The process and pressures of litigation are such that it is nearly impossible to escape its learning consequences and adverse effects on your pain problem. Think it over carefully.

Tension

Muscular tension and anxiety are well known as causes and aggravators of pain. While they are not synonymous and one can exist without the other, the two conditions often go hand-in-hand.

Do you think of yourself as a tense or anxious person? Consider whether or not you have any of the following symptoms: muscle tightness and soreness in the neck or shoulder areas, tension headaches, dizziness, rapid heartbeat, difficulty getting your breath, feelings of tightness in your chest or trembling hands? Do you worry too much, obsess over minor problems, have trouble relaxing or find yourself unable to put worries out of your mind when it's time to sleep? If you have any of the above symptoms, tension could be aggravating or even causing your pain problem. (If you haven't already done so, be sure to report any of these symptoms to your doctor since, in some cases, they may be related to other medical problems that should be treated.)

If you are tense or anxious, learning a technique known as 'progressive muscle relaxation' could be a big help to you. Properly practised and applied, it can help you to learn to relax quickly and effectively and even help you avoid becoming anxious in the first place. Chapter 10 discussed some abbreviated relaxation procedures to practise for pain caused by tension in a few specific muscles. Progressive muscle relaxation involves essentially the same procedures, but applied more completely and systematically to the whole body. It can be fun to learn and enjoyable to practise. Relaxation training, however, is like any skill. You become much better with practice. The ultimate aim is to prevent yourself from becoming tense and anxious and, in effect, change the way in which you respond to life's problems. Specific instructions on how to do progressive muscle relaxation can be found in Gerald M. Rosen's *The Relaxation Book: An Illustrated Self-Help Program*. If tension or anxiety is a problem for you, it could be worth your while to find and read a copy of this book. Relaxation training can also be learned from most psychologists. Call your local Pain Clinic or general practitioner for a referral to someone who can work on these exercises with you.

Summary

Any number of problems can co-exist with chronic pain. Some of the more common have been discussed here: sexual, relationship, social skills, assertiveness, failure to meet expectations, unhappy work situations, alcohol, litigation and tension. Through interaction, these things can aggravate a pain problem either by compounding it or by allowing the pain to serve the function of helping to avoid facing such other problems. The above list is by no means exhaustive. Any life problem can interact with pain. The important thing is to recognize what other problems may exist and to seek to change and correct them as part of your self-help programme. You can consult the 'Further Reading' section on pages 189–201 for self-help texts beyond the ones mentioned in this chapter. Seeking therapy can also be a means of solving such problems. Psychologists or social workers can be contacted through your local Pain Clinic (see Appendix), your GP or social services department.

Solution of other problems is especially important for the chronic pain sufferer. If you don't work on your other problems first or at the same time, the self-help procedures in this book will probably not work. Other problems interacting with the pain will be constantly working against your rehabilitation. However, provided you are willing to put in the effort, the right solutions to problems can almost always be found.

12. Maintaining Your Progress

The amount of improvement you can expect to achieve is hard to estimate in advance. The only way to find out how you respond to these procedures is to try them. They certainly won't work if you don't try them. Many former patients have indicated that, at first, they were very uncertain about the procedures, but they were willing to try them. They were pleasantly surprised when the techniques *did* work.

The goals of this programme can be broadly classified as learning to lead a more active, normal life, and reducing the importance of pain in your life. If you are to maintain whatever gains you may have made after your self-help programme, you first need to evaluate your progress in these areas. There are three possibilities:

1. you may not have improved at all,
2. you may have improved somewhat, or
3. you may have improved greatly. If you haven't met any of your goals for improvement, it may be that, in your case, a self-help book is not enough.

Some people need the help of a professional with whom they can work through the problems, brainstorm and discuss procedures, and who can reinforce their effort. The introductory chapters suggested that your doctor might wish to read this book with you and help you work on its programmes. Pain Clinics are also listed in the Appendix of this book so that you might consult them for help. Some clinics have outpatient programmes; others have inpatient programmes in which you can follow procedures similar to those outlined here but in a structured environment and with the help of many professionals. And, as mentioned earlier, a local psychologist may also be of assistance to you.

If you have made at least some progress through the use of this book, it will be important that you maintain that progress and not get re-caught in the Chronic Pain Trap. Remember that your problem is a *chronic* one. Chronic problems do not get cured, but they can be controlled. You will have to keep practising your techniques: thought-stopping, thought-switching, planning activities, self-reinforcement, relaxation, not discussing pain with others and so on. These actions and ways of thinking will need to become part of you *and* your family. They must be *continually* practised to continue working. This isn't as tedious as it sounds. With enough practice, they become quite automatic. And it is certainly less tedious than having chronic pain. If the techniques have helped you make some progress, practice will undoubtedly help you continue to make gains.

If your improvement has been dramatic, there is no less need to keep practising your exercises and techniques. Of course, living a more normal lifestyle is in itself more rewarding. The new behaviours you have learned may be maintained simply because they give you a fuller and more satisfying life. More healthy behaviour provides you with growth-oriented opportunities. New possibilities for life satisfaction are allowed to emerge. But certain maintenance activities are still a good idea for ensuring that all your improvement will last.

It is a good idea to check your progress at least once a month on a **Progress Report** (see page 185). If you can answer 'yes' to all of the questions on this worksheet, you are

Progress Report

Answer 'yes' or 'no' to the following questions to keep track of your progress. If you answer 'no' to any question, refer to the chapter indicated.

1. Are you fairly active every day? **(Chapter 5)** _____

2. If you are on medication, are you taking it on a regular schedule? **(Chapter 7)** _____

3. Have you been able to avoid increasing your intake of medication? **(Chapter 7)** _____

4. Are you successful at avoiding thoughts about pain? **(Chapter 8)** _____

5. Are you successful at avoiding conversation about pain? **(Chapter 8)** _____

6. Are you successful at avoiding showing pain? **(Chapter 8)** _____

7. Do you get dressed every morning? **(Chapter 8)** _____

8. Can you walk reasonable distances? **(Chapter 5)** _____

9. Can you sit for reasonable amounts of time? **(Chapter 5)** _____

10. Are you managing to keep pain from interfering with all the activities that you want to do? **(Chapter 5)** _____

11. Does your family successfully avoid discussing your pain or other problems? **(Chapter 9)** _____

12. Have you been regularly scheduling and enjoying pleasant events? **(Chapter 6)** _____

13. Are you trying to self-reinforce or praise yourself daily? **(Chapter 6)** _____

14. If your problem is a muscle tension one, do you practise relaxation often? **(Chapter 10)** _____

15. Are you using stress inoculation procedures regularly? **(Chapter 8)** _____

16. Have you solved or are you working on solutions to other problems which might aggravate your pain? **(Chapter 11)** _____

probably doing a good job of maintaining your progress. If you answer 'no' to any, return to the relevant section, re-read it and follow the procedures outlined anew. Occasionally have your partner or another family member give you his opinion of your progress by filling out the **Progress Report** for you. This can provide you with a more objective rating of your success and

Example Maintenance Checklist

List below the procedures or techniques from this self-help book which you have adopted and wish to remind yourself to practise as well as the frequency of your practice times, where appropriate. For each day of the week, check off whether you have used the procedure or technique as you had hoped.

Behaviours	Dates						
	16/3 Mon	17/3 Tues	18/3 Wed	19/3 Thur	20/3 Fri	21/3 Sat	22/3 Sun
Pain Cocktail							
8·00	✓	✓	✓	✓	✓	✓	✓
1·00	✓	✓	✓	✓		✓	✓
6·00	✓	✓	✓	✓	✓	✓	✓
Relaxation Exercises	✓	✓			✓	✓	✓
Walking ½ km / day	✓	✓	✓	✓	✓	✓	✓
Self-praise (read cards 2×/ day)		✓ ✓	✓ ✓	✓		✓ ✓	✓ ✓
Did not mention pain	✓	✓	✓		✓	✓	✓

serve to remind your family of its responsibilities in helping maintain your progress.

You can also develop your own **Maintenance Checklist** like the one shown below. Write down the key elements of the programme which you think worked for you and then check daily to make sure that you have followed them.

Maintenance Checklist

List below the procedures or techniques from this self-help book which you have adopted and wish to remind yourself to practise as well as the frequency of your practice times, where appropriate. For each day of the week, check off whether you have used the procedure or technique as you had hoped.

Behaviours	Dates						

The principles outlined in this book must be applied to the individual aspects of you and your lifestyle and working out how to do this is up to you. Only you can help yourself. Only you can take responsibility for controlling your pain. No one can do it for you. This book has provided you with some suggestions for techniques which many other people have found helpful. You will only know whether they work for you by trying them. And, if they do work, they will only continue working if you continue practising them and monitoring your progress.

Throughout the book you have been referred to as a 'pain patient'. But if you have read, absorbed and practised the programme in the preceding chapters, you should no longer need to think of yourself as a *patient*. You are no longer passively expecting help from someone. You are now actively providing yourself with help and coping strategies. You are controlling your chronic pain and making your life a much more satisfying experience.

Further Reading— For General Readers

Alcohol Problems

MILLER, W. R. and MUNOZ, R. F. *How to Control Your Drinking*. Prentice-Hall, Englewood Cliffs, NJ, 1976.

Assertive Problems

BOLTON, ROBERT H. *People Skills: How to Assert Yourself, Listen to Others and Resolve Conflicts*. Prentice-Hall, Hemel Hempstead, 1979.

DYER, WAYNE W. *Pulling Your Own Strings*. Hamlyn, London, 1980.

FENSTERHEIM, H. and BAER, J. *Don't Say Yes When You Want to Say No*. Futura, London, 1976.

JABERBOWSKI, PATRICIA and LANGE, ARTHUR J. *The Assertive Option: Your Rights and Responsibilities*. Research Press, Champaign, Illinois, 1978.

POWELL, JOHN. *Why Am I Afraid to Tell You Who I Am?* Fontana, London, 1975.

SHAW, MALCOLM E., WALLACE, EMMET and LABELLA, FRANCES N. *Making It Assertively*. Prentice-Hall, Hemel Hempstead, England, 1980.

SMITH, M. J. *When I Say No, I Feel Guilty*. Bantam Books, London, 1976.

Being Yourself/Liking Yourself

ELKINS, DON PERETZ. *Glad to Be Me: Building Self-Esteem in Yourself and Others*. Prentice-Hall, Hemel Hempstead, 1977.

LOUDIN, JO. *Act Yourself: Stop Playing Roles and Unmask Your True Feelings*. Prentice-Hall, Hemel Hempstead, 1980.

SKYNNER, ROBIN AND CLEESE, JOHN. *Families and How to Survive Them*. Methuen, London, 1983.

TWERSKI, ABRAHAM. *Like Yourself: And Others Will Too*. Prentice-Hall, Hemel Hempstead, 1979.

Change

BAKER, SAMM SINCLAIR. *Conscious Happiness: How to Get the Most Out of Living*. Bantam Books, London, 1976.

CALHOUN, L. G., SELBY, J. W. and KING, E. *Dealing With Crises: A Guide to Critical Life Problems*. Prentice-Hall, Hemel Hempstead, 1977.

DYER, W. W. *Your Erroneous Zones*. Sphere, London, 1977.

ELLIS, A. and HARPER, R. A. *A New Guide to Rational Living*. Prentice-Hall, Hemel Hempstead, 1975.

FREEMAN, LUCY. *The Sorrow and the Fury: Overcoming Hurt and Loss from Childhood to Old Age*. Prentice-Hall, Englewood Cliffs, NJ, 1978.

GOLDSTEIN, ARNOLD P., SPRAFHIM, ROBERT P. and GERSHAW, N. JANE. *I Know What's Wrong, But I Don't Know What To Do About It*. Prentice-Hall, Hemel Hempstead, 1979.

MAHONEY, MICHAEL J. *Self-change Strategies for Solving Personal Problems*. Norton, New York, 1979.

MAULTSBY, MAXIE C. JR. *Help Yourself to Happiness: Through Rational Self-Counseling*. Marlborough House, Boston, Massachusetts, 1975.

NEWMAN, MILDRED and BERKOWITZ, BERNARD. *How to Take Charge of Your Life*. Bantam Books, London, 1978.

VISCOTT, DAVID. *Risking*. Pocket Books, New York, 1978.

ZASTROW, CHARLES and CHANG, DAE H. (Eds.) *The Personal Problem Solver*. Prentice-Hall, Hemel Hempstead, 1977.

ZASTROW, CHARLES (Ed.) *Talk to Yourself: Using the Power of Self-Talk.* Prentice-Hall, Hemel Hempstead, 1979.

Depression

BURNS, DAVID. *Feeling Good.* New American Library, London, 1981.

LEWINSOHN, P., MUNOZ, R. ZEISS, A. and YOUNGREN, M. A. *Control Your Depression.* Prentice-Hall, Hemel Hempstead, 1979.

RUSH, JOHN. *Beating Depression.* Century, London, 1983.

Exercise

BOWERMAN, W. J. and HARRIS, W. E. *Jogging—A Medically Approved Physical Fitness Program for All Ages.* Corgi, London, 1971.

COOPER, KENNETH H. *The New Aerobics.* Bantam Books, London, 1970.

COOPER, MILDRED and COOPER, KENNETH. *Aerobics for Women.* Bantam Books, London, 1973.

DAVIS, ADELLE. *Let's Get Well.* Allen & Unwin, London, 1979.

DEVLIN, DAVID. *Your Good Health.* British Medical Association, London, 1978.

GETCHELL, B. *Physical Fitness: A Way of Life.* Wiley, Chichester, 1976.

JOHNSON, PERRY B. *Sport, Exercise and You · A Basic Textbook for Men and Women.* Holt-Saunders, London, 1976.

KERR, DAVID. *Cycling for Health.* British Cycling Bureau, London, 1977.

MAN, JOHN. *Walk! It Could Change Your Life.* Paddington Press, London, 1979.

MICHENER, LESLIE and DONALDSON, GERALD. *The Exercise Book.* Penguin Books, Harmondsworth, 1978.

PONTEFRACT, ROGER (Ed.) *Feel Fit, Come Alive.* Oxford University Press, Oxford, 1979.

TULLOH, BRUCE. *The Complete Jogger.* Pan Books, London, 1979.

Fears

MARKS, ISAAC M. *Living with Fear: Understanding and Coping with Anxiety.* McGraw-Hill, Maidenhead, 1978.

Controlling Chronic Pain

RACHMAN, STANLEY. *The Meaning of Fear*. Penguin, Harmondsworth, 1974.

ROSEN, GERALD. *Don't Be Afraid: A Program for Overcoming Fears and Phobias*. Prentice-Hall, Hemel Hempstead, 1977.

SMITH, MANUEL J. *Kicking the Fear Habit*. Bantam Books, London, 1978.

SUTHERLAND, E. ANN and AMIT, ZALMAN. *Phobia Free: How to Fight Your Fears*. Stein and Day, New York, 1977.

Leisure

GLASSER, RALPH. *Leisure: Penalty or Prize*. Macmillan, London, 1970.

LOCKE, ANTHONY. *Thinking About Leisure*. Ward Lock, London, 1968.

LOWEN, ALEXANDER. *Pleasure: A Creative Approch to Life*. Penguin, Harmondsworth, 1976.

RAPOPORT, RHONA and RAPOPORT, ROBERT N. *Leisure and the Family Life*. Routledge and Kegan Paul, London, 1978.

Marital

ADAM, J. and ADAM, N. *Divorce: How and When to Let Go*. Prentice-Hall, Englewood Cliffs, NJ, 1979.

BACH, G. R. and WYDEN, P. *The Intimate Enemy*. Avon, New York, 1968.

GOTTMAN, J., NOTARIUS, C., GONSO, J. and MARKMAN, H. *A Couple's Guide to Communication*. Research Press, Champaign, Illinois, 1976.

PAUL, JORDAN and PAUL, MARGARET. *Do I Have To Give Up All To Be Loved By You?* CompCare, Anapolis, Minnesota, 1983.

Pain

FORDYCE, W. E. *Behavioural Methods for Chronic Pain and Illness*. C. V. Mosby Co., St Louis, Missouri, 1976.

MELZACK, R. *The Puzzle of Pain*. Penguin, Harmondsworth, 1973.

STERNBACH, R. A. *Pain Patients: Traits and Treatment*. Academic Press, London, 1975.

Relationship

DIEKMAN, JOHN R. *Get Your Message Across: How to Improve Communication*. Prentice-Hall, Hemel Hempstead, 1979.

EGAN, GERALD. *You and Me: The Skills of Communicating and Relating to Others*. Brooks/Cole, Monterey, California, 1977.

GOLDSTEIN, HERB. *The New Male Female Relationship*. New American Library, New York, 1984.

JAMES, MURIEL and SAVARY, LOUIS M. *The Art of Friendship*. Harper and Row, London, 1978.

PECK, M. SCOTT. *The Road Less Travelled*. Hutchinson, London, 1983.

PRIESTLEY, P., MCGUIRE, S., FLEGG, D., HEMSLEY, V. and WELHAM, D. *Social Skills and Personal Problems: A Handbook of Methods*. Tavistock, London, 1978.

RUBIN, LILLIAN. *Intimate Strangers*. Fontana, London, 1984.

SATIR, VIRGINIA. *Peoplemaking*. Souvenir Press, London, 1978.

SHUTER, ROBERT. *Understanding Misunderstanding: Exploring Interpersonal Communication*. Harper and Row, London, 1979.

TEEAR, C. H. *Conquer Shyness*. A. Thomas, Wellingborough, 1977.

ZWELL, MICHAEL. *How to Succeed at Love*. Prentice-Hall, Englewood Cliffs, NJ, 1978.

Relaxation and Stress

ROSEN, GERALD. *The Relaxation Book: An Illustrated Self-help Program*. Prentice-Hall, Hemel Hempstead, 1978.

SELYE, HANS. *Stress Without Disaster: How to Survive in a Stressful Society*. Teach Yourself Books, Sevenoaks, England, 1977.

Sexual Problems

BERNE, ERIC. *Sex in Human Loving*. Penguin, Harmondsworth, 1973.

COMFORT, A. *Joy of Sex*. Quartet Books, London, 1978.

COMFORT, A. *More Joy of Sex*. Quartet Books, London, 1977.

GOCHROS, HARVEY L. and FISCHER, JOEL. *Treat Yourself to a Better Sex Life*. Prentice-Hall, Englewood Cliffs, NJ, 1980.

HEIMAN, J., LOPICCOLO, L. and LOPICCOLO, J. *Becoming Orgasmic: A*

Controlling Chronic Pain

Sexual Growth Program for Women. Prentice-Hall, Englewood Cliffs, NJ, 1976.

HITE, S. *The Hite Report.* Corgi, London, 1981.

HITE, S. *The Hite Report on Male Sexuality.* Macdonald, London, 1981.

Sleep Problems

COATES, T. J. and THORESEN, C. E. *How to Sleep Better: A Drug-Free Program for Overcoming Insomnia.* Prentice-Hall, Hemel Hempstead, England, 1977.

Women's Problems

FRIEDMAN, SUSAN, GAMS, LINDA, GOTTLIEB, NANCY and NESSELSON, CINDY. *A Woman's Guide to Therapy.* Prentice-Hall, Hemel Hempstead, 1979.

ORBACH, SUSIE and EICHENBAUM, LUISE. *What Do Women Want?* Fontana, London, 1984.

YATES, MARTHA. *Coping: A Survival Manual for Women Alone.* Prentice-Hall, Hemel Hempstead, England, 1977.

Work

BARTSCH, KARL and SANDMEYER, LOUISE. *Skills in Life/Career Planning.* Brooks/Cole, Monterey, California, 1979.

COOPER, GARY L. and PAYNE, ROY. *Stress at Work.* Wiley and Sons, Chichester, 1978.

LEVENE, MALCOLM. *The Second Time Around: Second Careers and How to Make Them More Successful Than the First.* Davis-Poynter, London, 1976.

References—
For Professional Readers

ANDERSON, T. P., COLE, T. M., GULLICKSON, G., HUDGENS, A. and ROBERTS, A. H. 'Behavior modification of chronic pain: A treatment program by a multidisciplinary team.' *Journal of Clinical Orthopedics*, 129: 96-100, 1977.

ARNOFF, G. M. and EVANS, W. O. 'The prediction of treatment outcome at a multidisciplinary pain center.' *Pain*, 14: 67-73, 1982.

ARNOFF, G. M., EVANS, W. O. and ENDERS, P. L. 'A review of follow-up studies of multidisciplinary pain units.' *Pain*, 16: 1-11, 1983.

BLOCK, A. R. 'Multidisciplinary treatment of chronic low back pain: A review.' *Rehabilitation Psychology*, 27: 51-63, 1982.

BLOCK, A. R., KREMER, E. and GAYLOR, M. 'Behavioral treatment of chronic pain: Variables affecting treatment efficacy.' *Pain*, 8: 367-375, 1980.

BOKAN, J. A., RIES, R. K. and KATON, W. J. 'Tertiary gain and chronic pain.' *Pain*, 10: 331-336, 1981.

BOND, M. R. *Pain: Its Nature, Analysis and Treatment*. Churchill-Livingstone, Edinburgh, 1979.

BONICA, J. J. *The Management of Pain*. Lea and Febiger, Philadelphia, 1975.

BONICA, J. J., LIEBESKIND, J. C. and ALBE-FESSARD, D. (Eds.) *Advances in Pain Research and Therapy: Proceedings of the Second World*

Congress on Pain. Raven Press, New York, 1979.

CAIRNS, D. and PASINO, J. A. 'Comparison of verbal reinforcement and feedback in the operant treatment of disability due to chronic low back pain.' *Behavior Therapy*, 8: 621-630, 1977.

CAIRNS, D., TZOMAS, L., MOONEY, V. and PACE, J. B. 'A comprehensive treatment approach to chronic low back pain.' *Pain*, 2: 301-308, 1976.

CARRON, H., DEGOOD, D. E. and TAIT, R. 'A comparison of low back pain patients in the United States and New Zealand: Psychosocial and economic factors affecting severity of disability.' *Pain*, 21: 77–89, 1985.

CATCHLOVE, R. and COHEN, K. 'Effects of a directive return to work approach in the treatment of workman's compensation patients with chronic pain.' *Pain*, 14: 181-191, 1982.

CAUTELA, J. R. 'The use of covert conditioning in modifying pain behavior.' *Journal of Behavior Therapy and Experimental Psychiatry*, 8: 45-52, 1977.

CHAPMAN, S. L., BRENA, S. F. and BRADFORD, L. A. 'Treatment outcome in a chronic pain rehabilitation program.' *Pain*, 11: 255-268, 1981.

DAVIDSON, P. O. (Ed.) *The Behavioral Management of Anxiety, Depression, and Pain*. Burner/Mazel, New York, 1976.

DOLEYS, D., CROCKER, M. and PATTON, D. 'Responses of patients with chronic pain to exercise quotas.' *Journal of American Physical Therapy Association*, 62: 1111-1114, 1982.

FEBREGA, H. JR. and TYMA, S. 'Culture, language and the shaping of illness: An illustration based on pain.' *Journal of Psychosomatic Research*, 20: 323–337, 1976.

FLOR, H. and TURK, D. C. 'Etiological theories and treatments for chronic pain. I. Somatic models and interventions.' *Pain*, 19: 105-121, 1984.

FOLLICK, M., ZITTER, R. and AHERN, D. 'Failures in the operant treatment of chronic pain.' In: E. B. Foa and P. Emmelkamp (Eds.) *Failures in Behaviour Therapy*. Wiley, New York, 1982.

FORDYCE, W. E. 'An operant conditioning method for managing chronic pain.' *Postgraduate Medicine*, 53: 123-128, 1973.

FORDYCE, W. E. *Behavioral Methods for Chronic Pain and Illness*. C. V. Mosby, St Louis, Missouri, 1976.

References

FORDYCE, W. E. 'Behavioral concepts in chronic pain and illness.' In: P. O. Davidson (Ed.) *The Behavioral Management of Anxiety, Depression and Pain.* Bruner/Mazel, New York, 1976.

FORDYCE, W. E., FOWLER, R., LEHMANN, J. and DELATEUR, B. 'Some implications of learning in problems of chronic pain.' *Journal of Chronic Diseases*, 21: 179-190, 1968.

FORDYCE, W. E., FOWLER, R., LEHMANN, J., DELATEUR, B., SAND, P. and TRIESCHMANN, R. 'Operant conditioning in the treatment of chronic clinical pain.' *Archives of Physical Medicine and Rehabilitation*, 54: 399-408, 1973.

FORDYCE, W., LANSKY, D., CALSYN, D., SHELTON, J., STOLOV, W. and ROCK, D. 'Pain measurement and pain behavior.' *Pain*, 18: 53-69, 1984.

FORDYCE, W., MCMAHON, R., RAINWATER, G., JACKINS, S., QUESTAD, K., MURPHY, T. and DELATEUR, B. 'Pain complaint-exercise performance relationship in chronic pain.' *Pain*, 10: 311-321, 1981.

FORDYCE, W. E., ROBERTS, A. H. and STERNBACH, R. A. 'The behavioral management of chronic pain: A response to critics.' *Pain*, 22: 113-125, 1985.

FORDYCE, W., SHELTON, J. and DUNDORE, D. 'The modification of avoidance learning in pain behaviors.' *Journal of Behavioral Medicine*, 5: 405-414, 1982.

GOTTLIEB, H., STRITE, L., KOLLER, R., MADORSKY, A., HOCKERSMITH, V., KLEEMAN, M. and WAGNER, J. 'Comprehensive rehabilitation of patients having chronic low back pain.' *Archives of Physical Medicine and Rehabilitation*, 58: 101-108, 1977.

GUCK, T. P., SKULTELY, F. W., MEILMAN, P. W. and DOWD, E. T. 'Multidisciplinary pain center follow-up study: Evaluation with a no-treatment control group.' *Pain*, 21: 295-306, 1985.

HALPERN, L. 'Psychotropic drugs and the management of chronic pain.' In: J. J. Bonica (Ed.) *Advances in Neurology Vol. 4: International Symposium on Pain.* Raven Press, New York, 1974.

IGNELZ, R. G., STERNBACH, R. A. and TIMMERMANS, G. 'The pain ward follow-up analysis.' *Pain*, 3: 277-280, 1977.

JESSUP, B. A., NEUFELD, R. and MERSKY, H. 'Biofeedback therapy for headache and other pain: An evaluative review.' *Pain*, 7: 225-270, 1979.

KEEFE, F. J., BLOCK, A. R., WILLIAMS, R. B. JR. and SURWIT, R. S.

'Behavioral treatment of chronic low back pain: Clinical outcome and individual differences in pain relief.' *Pain*, 11: 221-231, 1981.

KHATAMI, M. and RUSH, A. J. 'A pilot study of the treatment of outpatients with chronic pain: Symptom control.' *Pain*, 5: 153-172, 1978.

KHATAMI, M. and RUSH, A. J. 'A one-year follow-up of the multimodal treatment for chronic pain.' *Pain*, 14: 45-52, 1982.

LATIMER, P. B. 'External contingency management for chronic pain: A critical review of the evidence.' *American Journal of Psychiatry*, 139: 1308-1312, 1982.

LEVENDUSKY, P. and PANKRATZ, L. 'Self-control techniques as an alternative to pain medication.' *Journal of Abnormal Psychology*, 84: 165-168, 1975.

LINTON, S. 'A critical review of behavioral treatments for chronic benign pain other than headache.' *British Journal of Clinical Psychology*, 21: 321-337, 1982.

LINTON, S. 'The relationship between activity and chronic back pain.' *Pain*, 21: 289-294, 1985.

LUTZ, R. W., SILBRET, M. and OLSHAM, N. 'Treatment outcome and compliance with therapeutic regimens: Long-term follow-up of a multidisciplinary pain program.' *Pain*, 17: 301-308, 1983.

MCNAIRY, S. L., MARUTA, T., IVNIK, R. J., SWANSON, D. W., ILSTRUP, D. M. 'Prescription medication dependence and neuropsychologic function. *Pain*, 18: 169-177, 1984.

MARUTA, T., SWANSON, D. W. and SWENSON, W. M. 'Chronic pain: Which patients may a pain-management program help?' *Pain*, 7: 321-330, 1979.

MECHANIC, D. 'Social, psychological factors affecting the presentation of bodily complaints.' *New England Journal of Medicine*, 286: 1132-1139, 1972.

MELZACK, R. *The Puzzle of Pain*. Penguin, Harmondsworth, England, 1973.

MENDELSON, G. 'Compensation, pain complaints and psychological disturbance.' *Pain*, 20: 169-177, 1984.

MERSKY, H. and BOYD, D. 'Emotional adjustment and chronic pain.' *Pain*, 5: 173-178, 1978.

MERSKY, H. and HESTER, R. N. 'The treatment of chronic pain with

References

psychotropic drugs.' *Postgraduate Medical Journal*, 48: 594–598, 1972

MERSKY, H. and SPEAR, F. G. *Pain: Psychological and Psychiatric Aspects*. Bailliere, Tindall and Cassell, London, 1967.

MOHAMED, S. N., WEISZ, G. M. and WARING, E. M. 'The relationship of chronic pain to depression, marital adjustment and family dynamics.' *Pain*, 5: 285-292, 1978.

NALIBOFF, B. D., COHEN, M. J. and YELLEN, A. N. 'Does the MMPI differentiate chronic illness from chronic pain?' *Pain*, 13: 333-341, 1982.

NEWMAN, R. I., SERES, J. L., YOSPE, L. P. and GARLINGTON, B. 'Multidisciplinary treatment of chronic pain: Long term follow-up of low back pain.' *Pain*, 4: 283-293, 1978.

PAINTER, J. R., SERES, J. L. and NEWMAN, R. I. 'Assessing benefits of the pain center: Why some patients regress.' *Pain*, 8: 101-113, 1980.

PECK, C. 'Overcoming the chronic pain traps through the use of behavioural procedures.' In: J. Shepard (Ed.) *Advances in Behavioural Medicine*, Cumberland College Press, Sydney, 1981.

PECK, C. and LOVE, A. 'Chronic pain.' In: N. King and A. Remenyi (Eds.) *Behavioural Health Care*. Harcourt, Brace and Jovanovich, Sydney, 1985.

PECK, C. and WALLACE, M. (Eds.) *Problems in Pain*. Pergamon Press, Sydney, 1980.

PHILIPS, H. C. and JAHANSHAKI, M. 'The effects of persistent pain: The chronic headache sufferer.' *Pain*, 21: 163-176, 1985.

PILOWSKY, I. 'Abnormal illness behavior.' *British Journal of Medical Psychology*, 42: 347-351, 1969.

PILOWSKY, I. 'The diagnosis of abnormal illness behavior.' *Australian and New Zealand Journal of Psychiatry*, 5: 136-138, 1971.

PILOWSKY, I. 'Dimensions of abnormal illness behavior. *Australian and New Zealand Journal of Psychiatry*, 9: 141-147, 1975.

PILOWSKY, I., HALLETT, E. C., BASSETT, D. L., THOMAS, P. G. and PENHALL, R. K. 'A controlled study of amitriptyline in the treatment of chronic pain.' *Pain*, 14: 169-179, 1982.

PILOWSKY, I. and SPENCE, N. D. 'Pain, anger and illness behavior.' *Journal of Psychosomatic Research*, 20: 411-416, 1976.

Controlling Chronic Pain

ROBERTS, A. H. 'The operant approach to the management of pain and disability.' In: H. D. Holzman and D. C. Turk (Eds.) *Pain Management: A Handbook of Treatment Approaches*. Pergamon Press, New York, 1985.

ROBERTS, A. H. and REINHARDT, L. 'The behavioral management of chronic pain: Long-term follow-up with comparison groups.' *Pain*, 8: 151-162, 1980.

SERES, J. L. and NEWMAN, R. I. 'Results of treatment of chronic low-back pain at the Portland Pain Center.' *Journal of Neurosurgery*, 45: 32-36, 1976.

SHANFIELD, S. B., HEIMAN, E. M., COPE, D. N. and JONES, J. R. 'Pain and the marital relationship: Psychiatric distress.' *Pain*, 7: 343-352, 1979.

STERNBACH, R. A. *Pain: A Psychophysiological Analysis*. Academic Press, New York, 1968.

STERNBACH, R. A. *Pain Patients: Traits and Treatment*. Academic Press, New York, 1974.

STERNBACH, R. A. (Ed.) *The Psychology of Pain*. Raven Press, New York, 1978.

STERNBACH, R. A. and RUSH, T. N. 'Alternatives to the pain career.' *Psychotherapy: Therapy, Research and Practice*, 10: 321-324, 1973.

SWANSON, D. W., SWENSON, W. M., MARUTA, T. and FLOREEN, A. C. 'The dissatisfied patient with chronic pain.' *Pain*, 7: 367-378, 1978.

TAN, S. Y. 'Cognitive and cognitive-behavioral methods for pain control: A selective review.' *Pain*, 12: 201-228, 1982.

TURK, D. C. and FLOR, H. 'Etiological theories and treatments for chronic back pain. II. Psychological models and interventions.' *Pain*, 19: 209-233, 1984.

TURK, D. C., MEICHENBAUM, D. and GENEST, M. *Pain and Behavioral Medicine: A Cognitive-behavioral Perspective*. Guilford, New York, 1983.

TURNER, J. A., CALSYN, D. A., FORDYCE, W. E. and READY, L. B. 'Drug utilization patterns in chronic pain patients.' *Pain*, 12: 357-363, 1982.

TURNER, J. A. and CHAPMAN, C. R. 'Psychological interventions for chronic pain: A critical review. I. Relaxation training and biofeedback.' *Pain*, 12: 1-22, 1982.

References

TURNER, J. A. and CHAPMAN, C. R. 'Psychological interventions for chronic pain: A critical review. II. Operant conditioning, hypnosis and cognitive-behavioral therapy.' *Pain*, 12: 23-46, 1982.

VIOLON, A. and GIURGEA, D. 'Familial models for chronic pain.' *Pain*, 18: 199-203, 1984.

WEISENBERG, M. (Ed.) *Pain: Clinical and Experimental Perspectives.* C. V. Mosby Co., St Louis, Missouri, 1975.

WEISENBERG, M. and TURSKY, B. *Pain: New Perspectives in Therapy and Research.* Plenum Press, New York, 1976.

Appendix: Directory of Pain Clinics

The following list of Pain Clinics was supplied by the Intractable Pain Society of Britain and Ireland. If you as a patient are interested in seeking treatment from one of these Pain Clinics, the best way to do this is to have your doctor contact them to find out whether they treat the type of problem which you have and how an appropriate referral can be made.

ABERDEEN Aberdeen Royal Infirmary
ABERGAVENNY Nevill Hall Hospital
ABINGDON Oxford Regional Pain Relief Unit
   Abingdon Hospital
ASHFORD *Kent* William Harvey Hospital
BANBURY Horton General Hospital
BANGOR Caernarvon & Anglesey Hospital
   Caernarvon & Anglesey General Hospital
BARNSTAPLE North Devon District Hospital
BASINGSTOKE Basingstoke District Hospital
BATH Royal United Hospital
BEBINGTON *Wirral* Clatterbridge Hospital
BECKENHAM Beckenham Hospital
BELFAST Ulster Hospital, Dundonald
   Royal Victoria Hospital
   Mater Infirmorum

BIRMINGHAM Selly Oak Hospital
  Dudley Road Hospital
  East Birmingham Hospital
  Queen Elizabeth Hospital
BLACKBURN Blackburn Royal Infirmary
BLACKPOOL Victoria Hospital
BODELWYDDAN *Clwyd* Ysbyty Glam Clwyd
BOSTON Pilgrim Hospital
BRADFORD Bradford Royal Infirmary
BRIGHTON Royal Sussex County Hospital
BRISTOL Bristol Royal Infirmary
  Frenchay Hospital
  Bristol Maternity Hospital
  Southmead Hospital
BROMSGROVE Hill Top Hospital
BURNLEY Burnley General Hospital
BURY ST EDMUNDS West Suffolk Hospital
CAMBRIDGE Addenbrooks Hospital
CANTERBURY Kent & Canterbury Hospital
CARDIFF University Hospital of Wales
CARSHALTON Sutton Hospital
CHELMSFORD Chelmsford & Essex Hospital
CHELTENHAM Cheltenham General Hospital
CHESTERFIELD Chesterfield and North Derbyshire Royal Hospital
CHICHESTER St Richard's Hospital
  Royal West Sussex Hospital
CHRISTCHURCH MacMillan Unit, Christchurch Hospital
COUNTY DERRY Coleraine Hospital
COLCHESTER Essex County Hospital
COVENTRY Walsgrave Hospital
CRAWLEY Crawley Hospital
CUMBRIA West Cumberland Hospital
  North Lonsdale Hospital
DERBY Derbyshire Royal Infirmary
DONCASTER Doncaster Royal Infirmary
DOVER Buckland Hospital
DUBLIN St Laurence's Hospital
DUDLEY Burton Road Hospital
DUMFRIES Dumfries & Galloway Royal Infirmary
DUNFERMLINE Dunfermline & Fife Hospital

DUNDEE Royal Infirmary
DURHAM Dryburn Hospital
EASTBOURNE Eastbourne District Hospital
EDINBURGH Western General Infirmary
ENFIELD Enfield District Hospital
EPSOM Epsom District Hospital
EXETER Royal Devon & Exeter Hospital
FALKIRK Falkirk District Royal Infirmary
FRIMLEY PARK *Surrey* Frimley Park Hospital
GILLINGHAM Medway Hospital
GLASGOW Southern General Hospital
   Gartnavel General Hospital
   Victoria Infirmary
   Royal Hospital for Sick Children
   Royal Infirmary
GLOUCESTER Gloucester Royal Hospital
GREAT YARMOUTH Great Yarmouth General Hospital
GRIMSBY Grimsby District General Hospital
GUILDFORD St Luke's Hospital
   Royal Surrey County Hospital
HARLOW Princess Alexandra Hospital
HASTINGS Royal Sussex Hospital
HAVERFORDWEST Withybush Hospital
HAYWARDS HEATH Cuckfield Hospital
HENLEY ON THAMES Sue Ryder Home, Nettlebed
HIGH WYCOMBE Wycombe General Hospital
HULL Hull Royal Infirmary
IPSWICH Ipswich Hospital
KETTERING Kettering General Hospital
KIDDERMINSTER General Hospital
KING'S LYNN Queen Elizabeth Hospital
KINGSTON ON THAMES Kingston Hospital
   Sutton Hospital
KIRKCALDY Victoria Hospital
LANCASTER Lancaster Royal Infirmary
LEEDS General Infirmary
   Headingley Medical Centre
   St James University Hospital
LEICESTER Leicester Royal Infirmary
LINCOLN Lincoln County Hospital

LIVERPOOL Centre for Pain Relief, Walton Hospital
  Whiston Hospital
LONDON St Bartholomew's Hospital, London EC1A 7BE
  Middlesex Hospital, London W1
  Guy's Hospital, London SE1 9RT
  Whipp's Cross Hospital, London E11
  North Middlesex Hospital, Edmonton, London N18
  Central Middlesex Hospital, London NW10
  Charing Cross Hospital, London W6 8RF
  Westminster Hospital, London SW1
  Royal Free Hospital, Hampstead, London NW3
  Edgeware General Hospital, Middlesex
  St George's Hospital, London SW17
  Hammersmith Hospital, London W1Z 0HS
  St Thomas's Hospital, London SE1 7EH
  National Hospital, London WC1 3NBG
  Royal Marsden Hospital, London SW3 6JJ
  St Stephen's Hospital, London SW10
  National Hospital for Nervous Diseases, London WC1
  Whittingdon Hospital, London N19
  University College Hospital, London WC1
  St Christopher's Hospice, London SE26 6DZ
  St Andrew's Hospital, London F3
  St Joseph's Hospice, London E8
  Queen Elizabeth Military Hospital, Woolwich, London SE5
  Kings College Hospital, London SE5
LONDONDERRY Altnagelvin Hospital
LUTON Luton & Dunstable Hospital
MAIDSTONE West Kent General Hospital
MANCHESTER Royal Infirmary
  Christie Hospital
  Wythenshawe Hospital ·
  Park Hospital
  North Manchester General Hospital
  Withington Hospital
MIDDLESBROUGH South Cleveland Hospital
  Withington Hospital
NEWCASTLE UPON TYNE Royal Victoria Hospital
NEWPORT St Woolds Hospital
NORTHAMPTON General Hospital

NORTH SHIELDS Preston General Hospital
NORWICH Norwich & Norfolk Hospital
NOTTINGHAM Nottingham General Hospital
   Nottingham City Hospital
   Nottingham University Hospital
NUNEATON George Eliot Hospital
OTLEY Wharfedale General Hospital
OXFORD Radcliffe Infirmary
   Churchill Hospital
PEMBURY Pembury Hospital, Kent
PERTH Royal Infirmary
PETERBOROUGH District Hospital
PLYMOUTH General Hospital, Freedom Fields
PONTEFRACT General Infirmary
POOLE General Hospital
PORTSMOUTH Queen Alexandra Hospital, Cosham
PRESCOT Hypnotherapy Clinic, St Helen's Hospital
PRESTON Royal Infirmary
   Royal Preston Hospital
READING Royal Berkshire Hospital
REDHILL Redhill General Hospital
ROCHDALE Rochdale Infirmary
RUGBY Hospital of the St Cross
SALFORD Hope Hospital
SALISBURY Odstock Hospital
SCARBOROUGH Scarborough Hospital
SHEFFIELD Northern General Hospital
   Dept. of Continuous Care, University of Sheffield Medical School
SHREWSBURY Royal Shrewsbury Hospital
SIDCUP Queen Mary's Hospital
SMETHWICK Midland Centre for Neurosurgery & Neurology
SOUTH SHIELDS Diagnostic Centre, General Hospital
SOUTHAMPTON Royal South Hants Hospital
   Centre for the Study of Alternative Therapies
   Aldermoor Health Centre
   Southampton General Hospital
ST ALBANS City Hospital
ST HELIER, JERSEY Viscountess Clifden Centre for Pain Relief
STANMORE Royal National Orthopaedic Hospital
STEVENAGE Lister Hospital

STOKE ON TRENT City General Hospital
    North Staffs. Royal Infirmary
STOURBRIDGE Wordsley Hospital
SUNDERLAND Sunderland District General Hospital
SUTTON Royal Marsden Hospital
SWANSEA Ty Olwen Hospice
SWINDON Princess Margaret Hospital
TAUNTON Musgrave Park Hospital
TETBURY Tetbury & District Hospital
TRURO Royal Cornwall Hospital
UPPER BATLEY Dewsbury Clinic, Staincliffe General Hospital
VALE OF LEVEN Vale of Leven District General Hospital
WAKEFIELD Pinderfields Hospital
WEST BROMWICH Sandwell District General Hospital
WEYMOUTH Weymouth & District Hospital
WIGAN Wigan Infirmary
WINCHESTER Royal Hampshire Hospital
WIRRALL Clatterbridge Hospital
WOLVERHAMPTON New Cross Hospital
WREXHAM Maewr Hospital
YORK York District Hospital

Index

activities   27, 29, 30, 33-8, 43, 46-
    88, 98, 100, 101, 128, 129, 133-7,
    140, 142, 145, 147-51, 167, 185
    diary   30-3, 49, 51, 56, 57, 67,
        73
    levels of   14-17, 30-3, 38, 46, 47
    pleasant   98-107, 109, 147-51,
        165, 185
    recreational   15, 78, 79, 87, 100,
        101, 147-51, 192
    (*see also* exercises)
aggressiveness   96, 169
alcohol problems/dependence   4,
    27, 28, 163, 176-8, 181, 189
Alcoholics Anonymous   178
analgesics
    (*see* medication)
anger/resentment   4, 7, 20-2, 27-9,
    41, 136, 137, 161, 170, 176, 179
anorgasmic
    (*see* non-orgasmic)
anxiety   4, 9, 22, 97, 162, 164,
    175, 176, 180, 181, 191, 192
    social   96, 163, 169, 170

appetite, loss of   89
arguments   25, 26, 136, 167, 179
assertiveness   96, 97, 114, 169,
    181, 189, 190
attention   40-2, 44, 130, 138,
    142-4
attributes, positive   91-4, 174
aversive experiences   90, 95-8,
    109, 110
avoidance of problems
    (*see* denial)

baseline measurement   46, 48, 49,
    55-7, 66, 67, 70, 75, 77, 83, 86,
    87
bed rest
    (*see* rest)
behavioural medicine   43, 45
behaviour therapy
    (*see* counselling)
biofeedback   159, 160
    EMG   159
    thermal   159

blame   25, 26, 89

communication
  nonverbal   37
  skills   168, 169, 193
  verbal   37
compensation   16, 172-4
  (see also litigation, retirement,
    work)
complaining
  (see pain complaints)
complaint-resentment-guilt trap
  (see traps of chronic pain)
complications (of treatment)   7
conditioning effect
  of medication   1, 14, 114, 115,
    118, 125
  of compensation   16
  of family patterns   136, 139-52
  of other problems   162-82
contracting   46, 48, 50, 51, 56-61,
  66, 67, 69, 70, 72, 73, 74, 75, 77,
  78, 83, 84, 87, 99, 120-3, 127
conversation topics   145, 146, 150,
  151
coping statements   132, 133
counselling   164, 165, 168-70, 174,
  177, 178, 181
  marital   168
  sexual   164, 165
Crisis Centres   90
cues/reminders   48, 52, 56, 57,
  158

denial   22, 134, 137-40, 144, 161-
  82
depression   4, 16-18, 27, 29, 89-
  110, 134, 161, 191
  (see also helplessness, traps of
    chronic pain)
distraction   144, 166
doctors   26, 27, 28, 38, 39-45, 47,
  48, 78, 79, 87, 89, 112, 114, 120,
  122-4, 154, 160, 164, 178, 184

doctor-patient relationships   39-45
drug dependence   4, 11, 41, 118
  physical   11
  psychological   12
dyspareunia   164-6

effects on family   14-17, 17-22,
  134-52, 163-8
  (see also family patterns)
energy, lack of   27, 29, 89
excuses   57, 58, 60, 61, 69, 72, 74,
  150, 161-82
exercises   42, 46-88, 127, 130, 131,
  144, 191
  car riding/driving   46, 48, 50,
    73-8, 87
  housework   15, 47, 48, 79-84,
    87, 175, 176
  lifting   46
  sitting   48, 50, 66-70, 87, 128,
    147, 185
  stair climbing   46, 48, 50, 70-3
  stationary bicycle   46, 79
  tolerance   75, 77, 84
  walking   46, 48, 55-65, 87, 128,
    148, 185
  (see also activities)
expectations   40-2, 84, 94, 107,
  108, 123, 124, 130, 163, 170-2

faith in medical profession   5-9,
  27, 28, 39-41
family patterns   20, 22, 134-52
  (see also effects on family,
    responsibility)

fears
  (see anxiety)
fighting style   21
frontalis muscle   155

goals
  daily   46, 48, 50, 51, 53, 56-8,
    60, 61, 65-7, 69, 70, 72-5, 77,

78, 83, 85, 86, 87, 102, 120-3, 127
long-term 16, 107-9, 118, 138
graphing 51, 52, 59, 62-4, 66-8, 70, 71, 73, 76, 83, 87, 99, 127
guilt 4, 7, 12, 14, 18-21, 22, 27, 28, 29, 89, 91, 136, 137, 168

headaches 3, 5, 13, 14, 154-6, 159, 160, 165, 180
helplessness 89, 134
(see also depression, traps of chronic pain)
housework
(see exercises)
hypochondriac 3-9, 26, 27, 28

imagery 131-3
impotence 163-6
insomnia
(see sleep problems)
interest, loss of 89
internal dialogue 132
irritability 19, 111

learned pain
(see conditioning effects)
leisure
(see activities, recreational)
litigation 178-80
low back pain
(see pain)

maintenance of progress 183-8
checklist 187
malingering 6
(see also pain, imagined)
marital counselling
(see counselling)
marital problems 4, 7, 17-22, 28, 29, 163, 166-8, 181, 192
martyr 129
masseter muscle 155

medication 4, 10-14, 38, 40, 41, 43, 44, 89, 111-25, 130, 161, 176-8, 185
diary 115-17, 120
overdose of 13, 14, 17, 138, 178
record 112, 113, 115
trap 10-14, 27, 28, 41, 112, 114, 115, 178
monitoring, daily 46-88
mood elevation 47, 165
motivation 17, 27, 29, 51-3, 56, 65, 90, 122
muscular relaxation
(see relaxation)
muscular tension 22, 153-60, 180, 181, 185
forehead 154, 155
jaw 155, 156
neck and shoulder 156-8
muscular weakness 16, 47

neck/shoulder pain
(see pain)
nerve cocktail 124
non-orgasmic 164-6

overdose of medication
(see medication)
over-protectiveness 134-7, 140

pain 193, 194
attitudes 132
behaviour 128, 140, 143, 168
(see also pain complaints)
chronic syndrome 1, 2, 4, 5, 8, 11
Clinics 1, 2, 184, 202-7
cocktail 111, 118-25
complaints 19, 37, 43, 77, 140, 161, 167
(see also pain behaviour)
diagnosed 5
imagined 3, 4, 6, 8, 26-8, 43, 139

killers (*see* medication)
prevention of   153-60
rituals   130, 133
severe episodes   137-9, 140
talking about   131, 133, 144,
    184, 185
(*see also* pain, types of)
Pain Clinics
(*see* pain)
pain, types of
    abdominal   5
    facial   5
    limb   5
    low back   5, 14, 15, 17, 18, 55,
        66, 70, 137, 163-6, 170
    neck and shoulder   5, 154, 156,
        159, 176, 180
physiotherapist   48, 78, 87, 154,
    160, 170, 176
plans   146, 147
praise   59, 61, 73, 90-5, 97, 102-4,
    106, 107, 110, 133, 171, 172, 185
premature ejaculation   164-6
prevention of pain
(*see* pain)
progress
(*see* maintenance of progress)
psychologist/psychiatrist   7, 43,
    44, 90, 159, 160, 165, 168, 170,
    178, 181, 184
punishment   46, 48-61, 65-7, 69,
    70, 72-4, 77, 78, 83, 86, 87, 136,
    140

reciprocity   19, 20, 143, 168
recreational activities
(*see* activities)
rehabilitation   42-4, 146, 151, 179,
    182
    -facilitators   42-5
reinforcement
(*see* reward)
relaxation   129, 132, 153-60, 180,
    181, 184, 185, 193

resentment
(*see* anger)
responsibility   15, 20-2, 42, 45, 94,
    97, 109, 110, 123, 134-52, 187,
    188
(*see also* family patterns)
rest   33, 129, 140
    bed rest   15, 19, 127, 128
retirement   15, 29, 136, 172, 173,
    176, 179
(*see also* compensation, work)
reward/reinforcement   46, 48-61,
    65-7, 69, 70, 72-5, 77, 78, 83, 86,
    87, 90, 102-4, 109, 121-3, 129,
    140, 175, 179, 184, 185
    bonus   46, 59, 61, 67, 70, 73,
        75, 77, 102, 103
role change   43, 79, 136, 140-5,
    150, 151, 172-6, 190, 191
(*see also* family patterns, sick
    role, well role)
routine   129
(*see also* scheduling)

scheduling
    of activities   59, 61, 67, 73, 75,
        77, 78, 86, 98, 129, 130, 151,185
    of medication   114-25
    of relaxation   158
    of worry times   104, 105, 109
    (*see also* cues/reminders)
self criticism   59, 90, 91, 95, 96,
    172
self esteem   4, 16, 17, 28, 90-5,
    171-3, 174, 190
self image
(*see* self esteem)
sexual counselling
(*see* counselling)
sexual problems   28, 29, 163-6,
    181, 195
sick role   40, 42, 44, 126-33
(*see also* role change)
side effects of medication   114

sleep
  cocktail   124
  medication   17, 124
  problems   17, 89, 194
social anxiety
  (*see* anxiety)
social skills   169, 181, 193
  (*see also* anxiety)
social workers   181
stress inoculation   132, 185
suicidal thoughts   89, 90, 168
surgery   40, 41, 44, 167, 170, 176
swimming   79
sympathy   137, 168

take-it-easy trap
  (*see* traps of chronic pain)
task steps   80-3, 109
temporalis muscle   155
tension
  (*see* anxiety, muscular tension)
thought-stopping   91, 93, 95, 96,
  104-7, 127, 131, 143, 161, 184
tolerance, drug   11-14, 114
trapezius muscle   156
traps of chronic pain   4, 27, 28,
  29, 43, 44, 90, 140, 173, 176, 184
  complaint-resentment-guilt   18-
    22, 27, 29, 136
  depression   16-18, 27, 29

medication   10-14, 27, 28, 41,
  112, 114, 115, 178
take it easy   14-17, 27, 29, 46,
  47, 84, 136, 172, 176
treatment shopping   4, 6, 8, 27

understanding   24, 25, 27-9
  (*see also* sympathy)

vaginismus   164-6
vocational counsellor   174

walking
  (*see* exercise)
well behaviour   138, 144, 145
  (*see also* well role)
well role   126-33
  (*see also* role change, well
    behaviour)
work   196
  competitive   84-6, 172-6
  intolerable   163, 172-6
  loss of   16, 179
  part time   87, 174
  tolerance for   84-7
  volunteer   84, 85, 87
  (*see also* compensation,
    retirement)
worker's compensation
  (*see* compensation)